THE ULTIMATE GUIDE TO THE PHYSICIAN ASSISTANT PROFESSION

Notice

Medicine is an ever-changing science. As new research and clinical experience broaden our knowledge, changes in treatment and drug therapy are required. The author and the publisher of this work have checked with sources believed to be reliable in their efforts to provide information that is complete and generally in accord with the standards accepted at the time of publication. However, in view of the possibility of human error or changes in medical sciences, neither the author nor the publisher nor any other party who has been involved in the preparation or publication of this work warrants that the information contained herein is in every respect accurate or complete, and they disclaim all responsibility for any errors or omissions or for the results obtained from use of the information contained in this work. Readers are encouraged to confirm the information contained herein with other sources. For example and in particular, readers are advised to check the product information sheet included in the package of each drug they plan to administer to be certain that the information contained in this work is accurate and that changes have not been made in the recommended dose or in the contraindications for administration. This recommendation is of particular importance in connection with new or infrequently used drugs.

THE ULTIMATE GUIDE TO THE PHYSICIAN ASSISTANT PROFESSION

A PERSONAL MENTORING GUIDE TO SUCCESS

Jessica Rodriguez Ohanesian, MS, PA-C
Department of Emergency Medicine
Community Regional Medical Center
Fresno, California

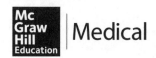

New York   Chicago   San Francisco   Athens   London   Madrid   Mexico City
Milan   New Delhi   Singapore   Sydney   Toronto

The Ultimate Guide to the Physician Assistant Profession

1 2 3 4 5 6 7 8 9 0   DOC/DOC   18 17 16 15 14 13

ISBN 978-0-07-180194-2
MHID 0-07-180194-4

This book was set in Plantin by Aptara, Inc.
The editors were Andrew Moyer and Peter J. Boyle.
The production supervisor was Catherine Saggese.
Production management was provided by Amit Kashyap, Aptara, Inc.
RR Donnelley was printer and binder.
This book is printed on acid-free paper.

Library of Congress Cataloging-in-Publication Data

Ohanesian, Jessica Rodriguez.
 The ultimate guide to the physician assistant profession : a personal mentoring guide to success / Jessica Rodriguez Ohanesian.

    p. ; cm.
 Includes bibliographical references and index.
 ISBN-13: 978-0-07-180194-2 (pbk. : alk. paper)
 ISBN-10: 0-07-180194-4 (pbk. : alk. paper)
 I. Title.
 [DNLM: 1. Physician Assistants.   2. Vocational Guidance. W 21.5]
 R697.P45
 610.73′72069–dc23

                                                            2013011583

McGraw-Hill Education books are available at special quantity discounts to use as premiums and sales promotions, or for use in corporate training programs. To contact a representative please visit the Contact Us pages at www.mhprofessional.com.

This book is dedicated to Jack, Dan, and Kristi.

Jack, being married to you is life's greatest blessing. I appreciate your love and support throughout this book writing process. Mom and Dad, thanks for your listening ear, support, and faith in what I can accomplish. I love you.

Contents

[CHAPTER 10]
Inspirational Leaders:
A Collection of Personal Professional
Biographies 253

About the Author

Jessica Rodriguez Ohanesian is a practicing physician assistant in emergency medicine. She has been a member of the American Academy of Physician Assistants (AAPA) and California Academy of Physician Assistants (CAPA) since 2005. She graduated from Western University of Health Sciences with a Masters Degree in Physician Assistant Studies in 2008. In the first year of her practice, she completed a one-year residency-training period in critical care, pulmonary, and sleep medicine. She lives in Fresno, California, and works at Community Regional Medical Center. Jessi finds inspiration in public relations opportunities and hopes to motivate and encourage those seeking more information about the physician assistant profession.

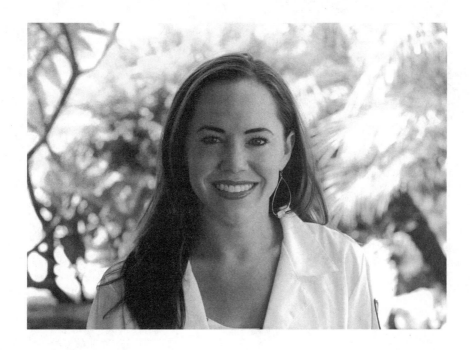

Contributors

Brynn C. Bailey-Van Sluis, MS, PA-C
Chapter 7: Endless Opportunities: Psychiatry

Christopher M. Barry, PA-C, MMSc
Chapter 7: Endless Opportunities: Pediatrics

Raj Bhatia, MD, FCCP
Chapter 6: Interprofessional Collaboration in Healthcare Delivery

Katie A. Boand, MS, PA-C
Chapter 7: Endless Opportunities: Orthopedic Spine Surgery

Sarah E. Broome, MS, PA-C
Chapter 4: Physician Assistant Student Life: General Surgery PA Student
    Rotation
Chapter 9: Incentive

Michael D. Burg, MD, FACEP
Chapter 6: Interprofessional Collaboration in Healthcare Delivery

Louise Capellupo, MS, PA-C, D-ABMDI
Chapter 8: Working Outside the Box: Forensics

Todd J. Doran, MS, PA-C, DFAAPA
Chapter 7: Endless Opportunities: Urology

Patrick F. Freeman. MHA, MMS, PA-C
Chapter 7: Endless Opportunities: Occupational Medicine and Urgent Care

Monika Fuller, PA-C
Chapter 7: Endless Opportunities: Bariatric Medicine

Wanda C. Hancock, MHSA, PA-C
Chapter 7: Endless Opportunities: Urology Female Perspective

Daniel Hestehauge, PA-S
Chapter 4: Physician Assistant Student Life: Didactic Year

Sarah Esther Hwang, MPAP, PA-C
Chapter 7: Endless Opportunities: Procedural PA in the Emergency
  Department Setting

Azita Javdanfar, MS, PA-C
Chapter 8: Working Outside the Box: Administration

Holly Jodon, MPAS, PA-C
Chapter 7: Endless Opportunities: Endocrine

Kristina P. Marsack, MS, PA-C
Chapter 7: Endless Opportunities: Plastic Surgery

Casey L. McCollum, MS, PA-C
Chapter 4: Physician Assistant Student Life: General Surgery PA Student
  Rotation

Daniel B. McConnell, MS, PA-C
Chapter 4: Physician Assistant Student Life: Summary of Clinical
  Rotations

José C. Mercado, MMS, PA-C
Chapter 7: Endless Opportunities: Otorhinolaryngology (ENT)

Michael P. Merren, MSM, MMSc, PA-C, AA-C
Chapter 8: Working Outside the Box: Anesthesiology Assistant and PA

Jessica Rodriguez Ohanesian, MS, PA-C
Chapter 1: History of the Profession
Chapter 2: Physician Assistants in the Healthcare System
Chapter 3: Physician Assistant School
Chapter 4: Physician Assistant Student Life: Introduction
Chapter 5: Transition from School to Work
Chapter 6: Interprofessional Collaboration in Healthcare Delivery:
  Introduction
Chapter 7: Endless Opportunities: Pulmonary, Sleep and Critical Care PA
  Residency and Emergency Medicine (published in *JAAPA*, June 2011)
Chapter 10: Inspirational Leaders: Personal Professional Biographies of
  Andrew Rodican, PA-C, William Kohlhepp, DHSc, PA-C, and Robert
  Sammartano, PA-C

Natasha Ohta, PA-S
Chapter 8: Working Outside the Box: National Health Service Corps
  Scholarship Recipient

Elizabeth Poss, MPAS, PA-C
Chapter 4: Physician Assistant Student Life: Pediatric PA Student Rotation

Lindsey Roberts, PA-S
Chapter 9: Incentive

Parisa Shabanzadeh, MPA, BA
Chapter 9: Incentive

Nesyah Shaesteh, PA-S
Chapter 9: Incentive

Jonathan E. Sobel, PA-C, FAPACVS, MBA
Chapter 7: Endless Opportunities: Cardiothoracic Surgery

Susanne J. Spano, MD, FACEP
Chapter 6: Interprofessional Collaboration in Healthcare Delivery

Breanne Strenkowski, PA-S
Chapter 9: Incentive

Rais Vohra, MD, FACEP, FACMT
Chapter 6: Interprofessional Collaboration in Healthcare Delivery

Tammy S. Woo, MPAS, PA-C
Chapter 7: Endless Opportunities: Family Practice

Previously published selections written by the following are republished in the book with permission from the American Academy of Physician Assistants (AAPA) and the *Journal of the American Academy of Physician Assistants* (JAAPA).

Robert G. Baeten II, MCMS, PA-C
Chapter 7: Endless Opportunities: Cardiac Critical Care (published in *JAAPA*, April 2011)

Scott Blow, MPAS, PA-C
Chapter 7: Endless Opportunities: Burn Center (published in *JAAPA*, December 2009)

Major Shawn T. Buller, APA-C, MPH
Chapter 8: Working Outside the Box: Aeromedical PA with the Army National Guard (published in *JAAPA*, April 2010)

Dawn Colomb-Lippa, PA-C
Chapter 8: Working Outside the Box: PA Professor and Orthopedic Clinician (published in *JAAPA*, June 2008)

Alexandra Godfrey, MS, PA-C
Chapter 4: Physician Assistant Student Life: Reality of Student Rotations (published in *JAAPA*, October 2009)

Pedro Gonzalez, PA-C
Chapter 8: Working Outside the Box: An Inspirational Entrepreneur (published in *JAAPA*, August 2006)

Catherine Hoelzer, MPH, PA-C
Chapter 8: Working Outside the Box: Missionary in Sudan (published in *JAAPA*, December 2006)

Laura Howard, MPAS, PA-C
Chapter 7: Endless Opportunities: Hematology: Renee Wittenmyer (published in *JAAPA*, October 2008)

Barbara Kimmons, PA-C
Chapter 7: Endless Opportunities: Obstetrics and Urogynecology (published in *JAAPA*, August 2005)

Nanette Laufik, PA-C
Chapter 8: Working Outside the Box: Queensland, Australia, PA
  Integration (published in *JAAPA*, February 2010)

Nicholas Oravetz, PA-C
Chapter 7: Endless Opportunities: Interventional Radiology (published in
  JAAPA, October 2007)

Jared R. Pennington, PA-C, MHS
Chapter 7: Endless Opportunities: Transplant Surgery (published in
  JAAPA, June 2006)

Shana Perman, PA-C
Chapter 7: Endless Opportunities: Neonatal Intensive Care Unit
  (published in *JAAPA*, August 2009)

Janette Rodrigues, writer/editor, AAPA News
Chapter 10: Inspirational Leaders: Professional Biography of Joyce
  Clayton Nichols, PA-C (published in *PA Professional*, September 2010)

Alexandra Braunstein Scott, MS, PA-C, MPH
Chapter 8: Working Outside the Box: Clinical and Health Research
  (published in *JAAPA*, February 2010)

Stephen Steiner, PA-C
Chapter 7: Endless Opportunities: Dermatology (published in *JAAPA*,
  April 2008)

James M. Taft, PA-C
Chapter 8: Working Outside the Box: Clinical Practice and Research in
  Neurology (published in *JAAPA*, October 2006)

Rebecca Tinsman, RPA-C
Chapter 8: Working Outside the Box: Volunteering in Rwanda (published
  in *JAAPA*, March 2009)

Lynn Tyrer, PA-C
Chapter 8: Working Outside the Box: Family Practice in the United
  Kingdom (published in *JAAPA*, August 2005)

Kaatje van der Gaarden, PA-C
Chapter 8: Working Outside the Box: Orthopedics in London, England
(published in *JAAPA*, December 2011)

Kristin K. Will, MHPE, PA-C
Chapter 7: Endless Opportunities: Hospitalist PA (published in *JAAPA*,
August 2007)

Jeffrey Yates, MPA, PA-C
Chapter 8: Working Outside the Box: Civilian Tactical Medicine
(published in *PA Professional*, February 2012)

Preface

Growing up, I knew I wanted a stable career that brought satisfaction through serving others. Medicine has always intrigued me. During my teens and early twenties, I swam competitively and worked summers as an ocean lifeguard. This experience introduced exercise physiology and first-responder medical knowledge. I explored different career options by shadowing family members and friends. Nursing didn't particularly spark my interest, but firefighting, law enforcement, and physical therapy all remained considerations. I knew my likes and dislikes, but my career search seemed to be missing that *one* option that spoke to my heart and said, "This is for me." I had not yet heard of a physician assistant (PA).

A seemingly unfortunate yet providential experience led to my discovery of the PA profession. Fourteen years of competitive swimming came to an abrupt end my senior year of college because of an injury. This freed up 4 to 5 hours each day. I used this newfound time to explore potential careers. Having an interest in physical therapy, I walked into the nearest hospital and asked if I could shadow someone in that profession. Luckily, the hospital said, "Yes," and this opportunity introduced me to a wide array of health professionals, including PAs. I decided then to pursue the PA profession but found very few resources to guide me, which planted the seed to one day write this book.

The American Academy of Physician Assistants (AAPA) webpage was the best resource available, and I joined as a student member. I then applied, and was accepted, to the school of my choice: Western University of Health Sciences. Having graduated from college magna cum laude, I started PA school with much enthusiasm and excitement.

I soon realized the course load and academic expectations were much more than I could have ever anticipated. To say that I struggled during the first three months would be an understatement. It was difficult to keep up with the fast pace and medical terminology. All exams had an allotted time, and many I was unable to complete. During my undergrad education, I was an "A" student. Now I had a "C" average. I knew at that point that my effort, determination, and study efficiency would be tested like never before.

During those difficult first few months in PA school, I wished I had a real-life PA mentor, a book to impart guidance, or *something* to provide hope and encouragement and say, "Hang in there, it'll all be worth it." I needed a light in that dark tunnel of 10-hour classroom days, daily exams, and weekends camped out in the library. I began PA school the youngest in my class, barely hanging onto a "C" average, and uncertain if I would even graduate. In the end, I finished in the top 10 in my class of 92 students, with national board scores in the 99th percentile. This turnaround began when I realized that PA school is not undergrad, and the energy and focus required were tenfold. There was no backup plan, and failure was not an option.

My first step toward making a turnaround was to meet with a counselor at my school's testing center. He watched as I took practice tests and gave me guidance on test-taking skills. It was hard to make time for these appointments, but in the end it was a necessary step that I had to take. I also signed up for tutoring with a second-year PA student. We met for 6 hours every Saturday. My exam scores and confidence improved. Every minute of the day counted, and I had a disciplined and detailed study plan for each upcoming exam. After the national board exam, I reflected on how much I learned through the PA school process and made a commitment to help every PA student I possibly could.

Mentoring PA students has become one of my passions. I have been in close contact with a large group of aspiring PAs, and I love hearing their personal stories of how they came to know about the profession. Encouraging them through the rough parts of PA school comes naturally to me. I sincerely love being a PA, and I want others to understand that the rewarding career in the end is worth the difficult road.

Aside from the PA profession, I love to write. After 2 years working as a PA, I submitted my first excerpt for publication, "A Day in the Life" of an emergency medicine PA for the *Journal of the American Academy of Physician Assistants* (*JAAPA*). While preparing this excerpt, I scoured through all the previously published "A Day in the Life" articles. I thought, "What an excellent resource for aspiring PAs. This content should be reorganized and marketed in book format." From that point on I began writing letters to publishers and organizing the table of contents for this book. McGraw-Hill expressed an interest making this project possible.

Through networking, I have solicited advice from literally hundreds of PAs on succeeding in PA school, student rotations, and the transition from school to the working world. In Chapter 4 you can read the hour-by-hour account of life in PA school and clinical rotations written by PA students. Chapter 7 includes a sampling of the most popular PA subspecialties in the "A Day in the Life" of a PA format. If you have an interest in rare PA subspecialties such as forensics, anesthesia, or administration, read

Chapter 8. Chapters 4, 7 and 8 have italicized common medical terms with glossary definitions to aid students in learning medical terminology. In the last chapter you will be inspired by the biographies of top leaders in the PA community. This book will help you to excel in PA school, give you a broader understanding of the many facets of this profession, and encourage you to *be your best*. Set no limits on what you can accomplish as a PA.

—Jessica Rodriguez Ohanesian, MS, PA-C

Acknowledgments

My own PA knowledge, experience and opinions were not enough to construct a comprehensive physician assistant profession manuscript. This book became a reality when my author contributors volunteered their time and passion into creating their own Day in the Life excerpts. These excerpts, along with the previously published, copyrighted material granted permission to republish by the AAPA and JAAPA, made this anthology complete.

Special thanks to my supportive editors from McGraw-Hill: Andrew Moyer, Peter Boyle, Kirsten Funk, Catherine Johnson, Midge Haramis, and Amit Kashyap. I want to thank my co-workers at Community Regional Medical Center, and my family and friends who supported me throughout the book writing process. Especially the following people who dedicated a large amount of their time editing or listening as my ideas solidified: Daniel Rodriguez (dad), Kristi Rodriguez (mom), Angie Rodriguez (sister), Sandy Young (grandma), Jack Ohanesian (husband), Jane Goodall (friend), Carol Houk (co-worker), and Lisa Hendey (mentor).

[CHAPTER 1]

History of the Physician Assistant Profession

The Physician Assistant History Society highlights eight distinct evolutionary periods in the development of the physician assistant profession.

- The precedent events and prototype period (1650–1960), where a concept similar to the physician assistant (PA) profession dates as far back as the seventeenth century, when Peter the Great used German military medical assistants in the Russian armies
- The ideological period (1961–1965)
- The implementation period (1966–1972)
- The evaluation and standardization period (1973–1980)
- The incorporation period (1981–1990)
- The consolidation period (1991–2000)
- The expansion and integration period (2001–2010)
- The maturation period (2011 to the present)[1]

The trend for physicians to leave generalist medicine and specialize began in the 1940s during World War II, when many injured soldiers required a specialist's care. After the war, the need for orthopedic surgeons, plastic surgeons, and rehabilitation physicians grew. The administration of Medicare in 1965 granted generous reimbursement for specialists and therefore encouraged new graduates of medical school to specialize in a specific field of medicine rather than remain in general practice. Incentives also included increased salary, prestige, a higher military rank, new technology, and grants toward medical research projects. This movement away from specialized medical care toward specialization among physicians began to create the need for physician assistants.

Times of war required medics and military corpsmen to work alongside physicians overseas, and as a result, they gained years of hands-on medical experience. According to *The Physician's Assistant: A National and Local Analysis*, by Ann Suter Ford, approximately 30,000 medics were discharged every year from the service, and only one-third found positions in healthcare in the early 1970s.[2] The development of the PA profession helped to solve two separate problems: the national shortage of generalist physicians and the lack of employment for ex-military corpsmen returning home from war.

Growth of the U.S. population, known as the *baby boom trend*, further increased the need for generalist physicians. Charles Hudson, MD, saw a solution to the problem and published his idea in the *Journal of the American Medical Association* in 1961. He proposed a midlevel provider program to train Navy hospital corpsmen with prior experience. In 1964, Dr. Stead, head of the Department of Medicine at Duke University, used Hudson's ideas to create a two-year experimental program, and he recruited four military corpsmen.[2] In August 1965, *Reader's Digest* featured an article about the up-and-coming program prior to its formal sanctioning.[3]

In 1965, the Academic Committee of the American Medical Association (AMA), chaired by Andrew Wallace, MD, granted permission for Dr. Stead to introduce his program at Duke University Medical Center in Durham, NC. He treated his PA students similar to medical residents. They did didactic training first but quickly transitioned into seeing patients on hospital rounds.[2] During the course of this experimental first PA program, an article entitled, "More than a Nurse, Less than a Doctor," appeared in the September 6, 1966 issue of *Look Magazine*.[4] The article's title, "More than, Less than," caused problems for the PA students at the time. Founding president of the American Academy of Physician Assistants (AAPA), William Stanhope, PA, MS, stated, "We felt like we were walking around the halls of Duke with a target on our backs." The brewing questions at the time were, "How did you get here?" and "What are you going to do?" An unpleasant reality was that many PAs were spoken to in the third person. While looking at the actual PA, people would say, "What are those PAs going to do here?"[5] This period of time, referred to as the *ideological period*, introduced the PA concept to organized medicine and the public.[1]

The establishment of PA programs and PA organizations, the enactment of model legislation, and the establishment of accreditation and certification procedures took place during the *implementation period* (1966–1972).[1] On October 6, 1967, the first three PAs, Kenneth Ferrell, Victor Germino, and Richard Scheele, graduated from Duke University's PA program. All three stayed at Duke to work after graduation.[2] Ferrell worked for a pulmonary and allergy specialist for 20 years and then left clinical practice to work in Duke's Private Diagnostic Clinic to analyze medical reimbursement.[6] Germino remained at Duke for six years, focusing on lung disease prevention and, later, prevention of organ rejection after intestinal and liver transplant. He left Duke to become one of the first commissioned PA warrant officers in the U.S. Coast Guard. He traveled to the Artic and Antarctic for the National Science Foundation and earned numerous awards for lifesaving rescues as a search and rescue team member.[7] Scheele worked in endocrinology his first two years and then transitioned into working for a private-practice cardiology group. Ironically, he died of a heart attack in 1970 at the age of 31. Prior to his tragic death, Scheele helped to establish the American Association of Physician Assistants in 1968, which later became the American Academy of Physician Assistants (AAPA).[3]

Activated, agitated students organized to form the AAPA. The core and primary motivation behind the start of the academy was education. There was need for a "unified voice" spoken from a PA point of view, for the PAs, which would positively support PA educators, and better inform the public. William Stanhope approached Dr. Harvey Estes with the AAPA idea, and he graciously loaned him the $600 that was needed to make incorporation in North Carolina. The academy grew through the symbiotic relationship and support of the programs at the time; Duke, Oklahoma, Baylor, Yale, and George Washington (GW) universities. During 1968–1971, AAPA focused on building a membership base, building a unified educational model, and the turmoil and struggle of "who they were." The first formal board examination ended much of this confusion.[5]

After the success of this first prototypical PA program, four other models were developed within a four-year period of time. One such model was Medicine Extension (MEDEX), developed by Richard Smith, MD. His emphasis was to train and transition his graduates to work in medically underserved communities on the West Coast.[2] In 1969, the first class of 15 former military corpsmen was selected for MEDEX and began training at the University of Washington. In 1971, the Washington State Medical Practice Act was amended and passed, allowing PAs to practice under the supervision of a licensed physician.[8] Other models included a surgeon's assistant program by John Kirklin, MD, a four-year baccalaureate degree program by Hu Myers, MD, and the child health associate program by Henry Silver, MD.[9]

In 1970, the AMA's House of Delegates passed a resolution recognizing PAs, and Kaiser Permanente became the first health maintenance organization (HMO) to employ PAs.[10] The following year, training program guidelines were developed by the AMA's Committee on Allied Health Education and Accreditation in order to maintain consistency among PA programs. The AMA House of Delegates adopted "Essentials of an Approved Educational Program for the Assistant to the Primary Care Physician" in 1971. This allowed for the provision of funds for PA training, and dozens of new programs began. For early PA students with a vocational calling to medicine, failure was not an option. There was no alternative career. Most of the early PAs were men in their middle to late twenties who had seen firsthand the poor treatment of male nurses and the bias of medical schools toward students over the age of 26.[5]

The *evaluation and standardization period* (1973–1980) began with the first annual AAPA conference in 1973, held at Sheppard Air Force Base, in Wichita Falls, TX, with 275 attendees. That same year, the National Board of Medical Examiners administered the first certifying exam.[2] Thomas Piemme, MD, founder of the PA program at George Washington University and founding president of the National Commission on Certification of Physician Assistants (NCCPA), states that "1972 is arguably the most significant year in the history of the physician assistant profession. Growth was about to become explosive, the AAPA meeting took place, accreditation began, programs multiplied with funding of 45 programs (36 of them new programs), and the National Board of Medical Examiners authorized the formal examination of certifying physician assistants."[5] The AAPA became an official organization and established a national office in 1974. During this period, continuing medical education (CME) and recertifying examination requirements for the profession were established, and enactment of PA enabling legislation occurred in most states.[1] The acclaimed Sadler twins, founding president of the Physician Assistant Education Association (PAEA) physician Alfred Sadler and his twin brother Blair, a lawyer, collaborated together in public health service during this period. They helped to develop the credentialing process for PAs, coauthored the book, *The Physician's Assistant: Today and Tomorrow*, and started Yale's PA program.[5]

"PAs working in an HMO can provide 79 percent of care traditionally performed by primary care physicians at 50 percent of the cost" was the statistic that introduced the *incorporation period* in 1981. PA roles were expanded, and more PAs sought out jobs in specialty fields. During this time, Medicare Part B approved reimbursement of PA services, and PAs obtained prescriptive privileges in most states. The first edition of the *Journal of the American Academy of Physician Assistants (JAAPA)* was published and distributed in 1988.[1]

Navy, Army, and Coast Guard PAs were commissioned in 1991 and 1992 in the *consolidation period* (1991–2000). This period provided new opportunities as states revised legislation and PAs were increasingly being used in a variety of healthcare settings (Veterans Administration, military and federal healthcare institutions, and HMOs). The AAPA reported 28,500 PAs in active practice in 1997, and PAs were granted rights to prescribe medication in 40 states, as well as the District of Columbia and Guam. In 2000, and after 25 years of effort at the legislative level, Mississippi became the last state to enact legislation authorizing PAs to practice in that state.[1]

The profession celebrated its thirty-fifth anniversary during the *expansion and integration period* (2001–2010). This period reflected rapid growth in numbers, as a record high of 4,267 PAs took the National Board Exam in 2001, with a 91.5 percent pass rate, and the number of accredited PA programs surpassed 130. International interest in the PA model of a teamwork approach to healthcare grew, and British, Canadian, and Dutch representatives met with the AAPA at the annual conference in 2002. The cutback in resident physician hours opened further opportunities for PAs in hospital and inpatient settings.[1]

As of midyear 2012, there are "86,500 certified PAs" practicing in the United States.[11] We owe our gratitude to the first generation of PAs who fought for the profession at the legislative and clinical levels. Their pioneering efforts demonstrated the capabilities of a PA and established the legal foundation for this profession. The competence and professionalism with which they treated patients earned the confidence and trust of physician colleagues and patients alike.[12]

References

1. Physician Assistant History Society. *Honoring Our History, Ensuring Our Future.* Johns Creek, GA, 2011; available at: www.pahx.org/timeline.html.

2. Kent, A. "History of Service." *PA Professional*, September 2010.

3. Carter, R. "Richard J. Scheele, PA." In *Honoring Our History, Ensuring Our Future.* Physician Assistant History Society, Johns Creek, GA, 2010; available at: www.pahx.org/scheele-richard-j.

4. Carter, R. "Kathleen Gainor Andreoli, DSN, FAAN." In *Honoring Our History, Ensuring Our Future*. Physician Assistant History Society, Johns Creek, GA, 2008; available at: www.pahx.org/andreoli-kathleen-gainor.

5. Ballweg, R., Piemme, T., Sadler, A., Jr., and Stanhope, W. "The Way We Were: A Conversation with PA Profession's Early Leaders." Physician Assistant History Society, Johns Creek, GA. Recorded by LAVA Post Production, 2011.

6. Carter, R. "Kenneth F. Ferrell, PA." Physician Assistant History Society, Johns Creek, GA, 2010; available at: www.pahx.org/ferrell-kenneth-f.

7. Carter, R. "Victor H. Germino, Jr., PA-C." In *Honoring Our History, Ensuring Our Future*. Physician Assistant History Society, Johns Creek, GA, 2010; available at: www.pahx.org/germino-victor-h.

8. MEDEX Northwest Division of Physician Assistant Studies. Physician Assistant Training Program. Seattle, WA, 2011; www.washington.edu/medicine/som/depts/medex/whoweare/history.htm.

9. Piemme, S. "Regulatory History of the Physician Assistant Profession: History of Service." *PA Professional*, September 2010.

10. Physician Assistant History Society. "Implementation Period (1966–1972)." Johns Creek, GA, 2011; available at: http://pahx.org/period03.html.

11. Business Wire. "NCCPA Certifies 100,000th Physician Assistant." New York, 2012; available at: www.canada.com/business/NCCPA+Certifies+000th+Physician+Assistant/7295426/story.html.

12. Stanhope, W. "The First Generation of PAs." *PA Professional*, November 2011.

[CHAPTER 2]

Physician Assistants in the Healthcare System

According to research completed by the Business Networking Academy (BNA), 90 percent of people ask, "So, what do you do?" as their opening question on meeting a new business acquaintance.[1] As controversial and intrusive as this question is, many people use their occupation as a way to identify themselves and others. Forty hours per week, roughly 2,000 hours per year, are spent in one's chosen occupation. This chapter summarizes physician assistant prerequisites, training, supervision, and competencies. It also dissects the differences between nurse practitioners and physician assistants, and outlines the growth, pros and cons of the physician assistant profession.

WHAT IS A PHYSICIAN ASSISTANT?

A physician assistant (PA) is a licensed, nationally board-certified healthcare provider dedicated to patient care through team practice with and under the supervision of a licensed physician. There are currently 173 accredited PA programs in the United States.[2] The vast majority award master's degrees. PA education programs are represented by the Physician Assistant Education Association (PAEA) and accredited through the Accreditation Review Commission on Education for the Physician Assistant (ARC-PA). The average length of PA school is 27 months, and admission is highly competitive.[3]

Most PA programs have the following prerequisites: chemistry, anatomy, physiology, biology, microbiology, genetics, and statistics. Additionally, most PA programs require applicants to have prior healthcare experience.

The first year of PA school is didactic, or classroom learning. During the second year of PA school, students complete more than 2,000 hours of clinical rotations, with an emphasis on primary care, in physicians' offices hospitals or long-term care facilities. Most PA schools require rotations in family medicine, internal medicine, obstetrics and gynecology, pediatrics, general surgery, emergency medicine, and psychiatry. Schools often allow students to select electives in the specialty of their choice.[3]

Training to give outstanding patient care is the PA school's primary focus. Physicians and PAs are trained similarly using the medical model, which focuses on the physical and biologic aspects of disease. The duration of didactic and clinical training, however, is longer for a physician, and physicians are required to choose a specialty and complete residency training after medical school. The training of the two professions complements each other and improves accessibility to quality healthcare for patients. In addition, "the medical partnership between physician and PA multiplies the capitalization of the supervising physician's specialized skills, time and billing. PAs are cost-effective medical providers and contribute to the financial foundation of healthcare."[4]

On an individual basis, physicians supervising PAs define their scope of practice in a formal agreement called the *Delegation of Services*. This agreement is discussed and signed during the hiring process. A PA's duties commonly include evaluating, diagnosing, and treating new and existing medical and surgical conditions, initiating and interpreting laboratory and imaging results, performing minor medical and surgical procedures, assisting physicians in medical and surgical procedures, and writing prescription medications. Duties also include writing or dictating progress notes on patients' charts, performing follow-up patient care, providing health education to patients and families, referring patients for specialized consultations, and coordinating activities related to patient care within the clinic or hospital.

Four national PA organizations have united to define PA competencies. The organizations include the American Academy of Physician Assistants (AAPA), the Accreditation Review Commission on Education for the Physician Assistant, Inc. (ARC-PA), the National Commission on Certification of Physician Assistants (NCCPA), and the Physician Assistant Education Association (PAEA). The PA competencies are incorporated into the practice, training, continuing education, and evaluation of PAs.[5]

PHYSICIAN ASSISTANT COMPETENCIES

1. "Medical Knowledge is defined as an understanding of epidemiology, pathophysiology, diagnosis, management, and prevention of disease.

2. Interpersonal and Communication Skills are an important part in effective information exchange with patients, patient family members, members of the healthcare team and the healthcare system.

3. Patient Care is the ability to provide healthcare that is compassionate, appropriate, and effective for the treatment of health problems and the promotion of health across the life span.

4. Professionalism is a commitment to personal development, individual accountability, ethical practice, sensitivity to a diverse patient population, and adherence to legal and regulatory requirements in healthcare.

5. Practice-Based Learning and Improvement is an ongoing dedication to assess, evaluate, and improve patient care practices.

6. Systems-Based Practice encompasses the societal, organizational, and economic environments in which healthcare is delivered."[6]

HOW PHYSICIAN ASSISTANTS DIFFER FROM NURSE PRACTITIONERS

In 1957, registered nurse Thelma Ingles began a clinical sabbatical in an attempt to establish a master's degree program for nurses with Dr. Eugene A. Stead at Duke University. The program was a success with the school and the students but was denied accreditation by the National League of Nursing (NLN). Eight years later, Dr. Stead teamed up with registered nurse Kathleen Gainor Andreoli to revise the curriculum and educate the first class of PAs. Nurse Andreoli became the program's first academic coordinator and guided Duke University through the first five years of the program. Leaders of the American Nurses Association were initially skeptical of the PA concept. But the 1966 *Look Magazine* article, "More than a Nurse, Less than a Doctor," stimulated nurses toward the emerging nurse practitioner (NP) concept.[7] PAs and NPs were closely linked in the early years, so much so that they took the initial certifying examination together given by the National Board of Medical Examiners in 1973.[8]

Currently, both PAs and NPs are employed and have prescriptive rights in all 50 states. Each state has its own rules and regulations regarding supervision by a physician and limitations in prescription rights. There is often confusion over the differences between a PA and an NP because both are viewed as midlevel providers and both work in similar settings. Competition in the job market can occur, and some hospitals or clinics may favor one profession over another. PAs are seen as dependent providers, with a focus on the teamwork approach to medicine with their supervising physician. The teamwork approach is how the profession started and is believed to benefit all parties. NPs are independent providers in some states. The dichotomy between PA and NP practicing rights lies within legislation. Table 2-1 lists some of the key differences between PAs and NPs.

Table 2-1. Differences between Physician Assistants and Nurse Practitioners

	Physician Assistant	Nurse Practitioner
Training	Medical model	Nursing model
Prerequisites	BA or BS with any major required prior to starting most PA schools, with the exception of some bachelor-based PA programs	BS in nursing or "affiliated science" required prior to starting NP school
Time spent in supervised clinical rotations	9–15 months	(three semesters)
Foundational model for training	Trained as a generalist, with the flexibility to change/be trained in any subspecialty	Trained as a specialist in acute care, women's health, family health, or anesthesia; limited flexibility in changing subspecialties
Supervision requirements	Dependent practioners; a supervising physician is required for contract agreements in all states	Independent practitioners in some but not all states
Business opportunities	Can own a business but must hire a supervising physician	Can own a business in some states without a supervising physician

The medical model has been used since the time of Koch and Pasteur and is the traditional approach to diagnosis and treatment of disease. The basic sciences, pathophysiology, and disease presentation and treatment are taught prior to clinical experience. It is built on the physical and biologic aspects of disease and is *problem*-focused. Patient-related decisions are evidence-based.

The nursing model differs in its holistic approach to treat the whole person and is *patient*-focused. All dimensions of a person—mental, emotional, spiritual, and physical—are explored to find the cause of a problem. During training, the basic sciences are taught in conjunction with clinical rotations.

GROWTH OF THE PHYSICIAN ASSISTANT PROFESSION

"The Bureau of Labor Statistics predicts that PAs will be the second-fastest-growing profession in the next decade, increasing from 74,800 in 2008 to 103,900 in 2018. AAPA projects that in 2020, there will be between 137,000 and 173,000 certified PAs."[9] Figure 2-1 shows the growth curve since the 1967 when the first three PAs started.[8]

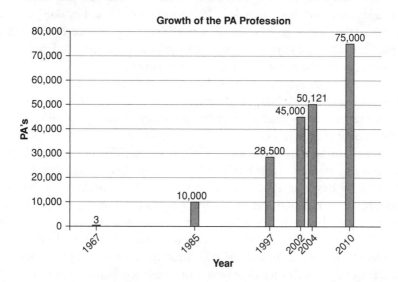

Figure 2-1. Growth of the physician assistant profession. (*Reproduced with permission from A. Kent, "History of Service," PA Professional, September 2010.*)

PROS AND CONS OF THE PHYSICIAN ASSISTANT PROFESSION

As with any other profession, advantages and disadvantages abound. A wide range of PAs contributed to this section by sharing their subjective opinions on this topic. The content highlights the main advantages and disadvantages of the life of a PA professional, and is designed to "tell it like it is" from a PA perspective. It is not intended to offend or discredit any other medical health professionals.

The Pros

In a market research survey in 2002, nine of ten PAs would choose the same career path if given the opportunity, and that job-satisfaction trend continues today.[10] The profession is unique in its design. PAs are both part of a team and yet autonomous to practice medicine. In many practice settings, PAs see patients unaided and consult with the supervising physician as needed or at the patient's request. Each workday reveals new patient challenges and experiences. Flexibility and variety set PAs apart from any other profession in the medical field. PAs are trained in primary care, yet they have the option to work in a wide variety of the many subspecialties in medicine and can change course at any point. For example, a PA can practice obstetrics one year and psychiatry the next year. In contrast, a physician must choose a subspecialty in medical school, complete a three- to five-year residency, and remain in that specialty for the rest of his or her medical career.

As a PA, your academic adrenaline will surge as your knowledge base improves. Learning is perpetual. Every day is an opportunity to learn something new from your supervising physician, your colleagues, nurses, or the patients themselves.

PAs are in high demand, and the job is secure. The profession is more accepted and rapidly expanding as physicians are becoming more familiar with how to best use PAs. The profession is economically ideal because schooling is shorter and less expensive than medical school. PAs can start their career in the medical workforce 6 to 7 years after high school graduation, whereas it takes 11 to 17 years after high school for physicians to complete their education and training. Becoming a medical professional at a young age or in a shorter time span can be especially important for working mothers. After becoming a PA, there is ample time to gain experience, develop as a professional, and build financial security prior to starting a family. There is financial stability within the profession, and the average annual salary ranges from approximately $75,000 to $150,000 depending on work setting and geographic location.

PAs may have lower stress levels than physicians because they have less legal responsibility. Most PAs job duties focus on patient care, not on the business aspects of hiring and firing, billing and reimbursement, and marketing. PAs and physicians are both subject to lawsuits, but when a PA is sued, usually his or her attending physician provides guidance and support throughout the process.

As a healthcare provider, a PA is reminded daily about the importance of health, fitness, and well-being. Taking care of ill and obese patients provides sufficient motivation to schedule preventative health screening examinations and to maintain a healthy weight. Clinical experience helps a PA to understand when to seek medical or surgical attention regarding his or her own healthcare. PAs have a positive influence on others as they educate, counsel, and encourage people daily, and the ability to form relationships with patients as a healthcare provider is rewarding.

As a PA, you will have a stable career that brings satisfaction at the end of each day. You help people, learn from people, and each day is unprecedented. You have the flexibility to increase or decrease your work hours, change subspecialties, or switch to a non–patient care environment such as education, administration, or research.

The Cons

Introducing oneself as a PA might draw a confused or dissatisfied reaction. Your patient may be thinking, "What's a PA? Are you a nurse? How much information do I need to share with this person? Should I tell him the truth about why I am here and what I need? Should I ask to see a physician, too, or is she coming in later?"

Jennifer Nowaczyk, PA-C, gives a choice example of the frustrations of a patient's first encounter with a PA. "No, I am not a medical assistant. No, I am never going to go to medical school. No, I am neither a nurse nor a nurse practitioner." She warns, "Get used to it now. You will be teaching a lot of people what a PA is and what exactly we can and cannot do. Take pride in this conversation, and use it to educate people."

There are still medical colleagues who often do not understand or respect the role of a PA. Most physicians are respectful, but a select few are not. It could take several months or up to several years to prove yourself to a supervising physician or group of providers. Alternatively, physicians as a whole are respected because of their well-recognized, prestigious title and the extensive education they receive in comparison with a PA.

Scheduling can become a con. If you choose to work for only one physician, you will likely feel compelled to take vacation when he or she does due to convenience in patient scheduling. Often, in those circumstances, there is not another PA trained specifically to work with your supervising physician, so sick days or relief can become nonexistent. This is important to keep in mind when signing a job contract. Flexibility with scheduling and vacation time will correspond to the size of the practice and the number of PA coworkers.

PAs must stay within their scope of practice. There are limitations to what you can do. The PA and supervising physician sign a *Delegation of Services* and Protocols agreement together, and ultimately, the supervising physician dictates what procedures a PA can do and what medications can be prescribed. When there is disagreement between a PA and a physician about a patient's appropriate treatment, the physician makes the final decision. These aspects of the profession are important to consider when it comes to personality. The profession is a mismatch for those who may not be able to handle their job title not being understood or the idea that someone else has the authority to make the final decision. Suzie LeRoy, PA-C, warns, "You are not a doctor. If you secretly want to be one, then the PA profession is not for you."

I love being a PA, practicing medicine and making a difference. I would not change what I do. This does not mean that there are not days when I am frustrated, angered, or annoyed with being a PA. But I love the flexibility; I have worked the typical 40-hour week, and I have worked the nights/days/ weekends/holiday schedules. No matter what turn my life takes, I can find a PA job to fit it. I love that I can have a crazy day in the ICU, placing central lines, intubating, coding, and at the end of the day I go home, not to the office to start my administrative work. At the same time, there are days when I am used as more of an intern. This is not because my boss does not trust me, but when it comes down to the paper work, who do you really think is going to do it—the PA or the MD?

—Jennifer Nowaczyk, PA-C

I love my job and seeing patients. The versatility is attractive, and if you want to change specialties after a few years, it's very easy to do. The drawback of being a PA is that there are some occasions when you want to be independent and it is not possible. Being an NP [nurse practitioner], you can "hang out your own shingle" and be independent on some level, while this is not possible for PAs. There are some hospitals that also do not want to hire PAs because of logistics and the need for the supervising physician to be variable. PAs are required to register with only one supervising physician and then anyone in the group can be the secondary physician. With NPs, they can see patients for any group in the hospital.

—Rebecca Isaacson, PA-C

The PA profession is the best job in the world. I have the flexibility to work anywhere and in any discipline. It is easy to move around if I want to. It is still such a young profession and still unrecognized by many. The most frustrating aspect is turf wars with other medical professionals, which is a waste of time, when the real goal should be patient care. But even in the time I've been a PA, I have seen so many more medical professionals, the public, and even law makers become much more educated about the profession. As long as we continue to be professionals and deliver high-quality, compassionate patient care, we will continue to be recognized as an integral part of the healthcare delivery system.

—Cyndy Flores, PA-C, Director of PA/NP Operations, CEP America

Pros of the profession include the versatility to change disciplines, flexibility in scheduling, and job security. Cons include patients being unfamiliar with what a PA is, supervising physicians who are unsupportive, and the title of a PA being misunderstood as a medical assistant.

—Stephanie Hannah, MMS, PA-C

References

1. Adonis, J. "So, What Do You Do?" *Sydney Morning Herald.* My Small Business, 2012; www.smh.com.au/small-business/blogs/work-in-progress/so-what-do-you-do-20120503-1y277.htm.

2. Accreditation Review Commission on Education for the Physician Assistant, Inc. Accredited Entry-Level Programs. Updated April 12, 2013.

3. American Academy of Physician Assistants. "What Is a PA? How Are PAs Educated and Trained? www.aapa.org/the_pa_profession/what_is_a_pa.aspx.

4. Memorandum of Understanding Physician Assistant. Committed to Excellence in Their Medical Practice and Patient Care . . . Character and Value; www.paworld.net/contractissues.htm.

5. Physician Assistant Competencies: Online Center, 2006; www.nccpa.net/PAC/Competencies_home.aspx.

6. American Academy of Physician Assistants. "PA Competencies Key." *IMPACT: Explore the Possibilities*. General information handout, Toronto, Canada, 2012, p. 17.

7. Carter, R. "Kathleen Gainor Andreoli, DSN, FAAN." In *Honoring Our History, Ensuring Our Future*. Physician Assistant History Society, Johns Creek, GA, 2008; available at: www.pahx.org/andreoli-kathleen-gainor.

8. Kent, A. "History of Service." *PA Professional*, September 2010.

9. American Academy of Physician Assistants. "Past, Present and Future: What Are Projections for the Future Growth of the Profession? And Why Is It Growing SO Fast? Available at: www.aapa.org/the_pa_profession/quick_facts/resources/item.aspx?id=3840.

10. Physician Assistant History Society. *Honoring Our History, Ensuring Our Future*. Johns Creek, GA, 2011; available at: www.pahx.org/timeline.html.

[CHAPTER 3]

Physician Assistant School

This chapter is designed for current or prospective physician assistant (PA) students.* It covers the didactic, or baseline knowledge, portion of PA school. For most schools across the nation, the first year of the program involves eight-hour classroom days, five days a week, for a year, with biweekly examinations. Be aware, it is accelerated. A more pleasant didactic course of PA school is guaranteed to those students who are properly prepared and aware of what to expect. The material in this chapter addresses financial concerns, coursework load, study tips, time management, and necessary support systems during PA school.

FINANCIAL PREPAREDNESS

A PA educational program is expensive. Across the country, the average tuition cost of a PA program is $50,000. Cost varies depending on the length of the program, whether the school is private or public, and whether you are an in-state or out-of-state resident. Paying for school can be an ominous task.

There are multiple financial aid opportunities available to students. Take some time to learn about your options, and apply early. An impor-

---

*If you have not yet been accepted to a PA program, consider these resources: *The Ultimate Guide to Getting into Physician Assistant School*, by Andrew Rodican, PA-C, gives insight for selecting a program, completing the application, writing an essay, and nailing the interview. His second book, *How to "Ace" the Physician Assistant School Interview*, will help you to master interview strategies, develop your selling-proposition statement, and prepare answers for potential interview questions.

tant preliminary step for this process is to complete and submit the Free Application for Federal Student Aid (FAFSA).[1] Financial aid counselors recommend submitting your FAFSA early, even if you have not been formally accepted to any PA school. After your FAFSA has been processed, the schools that have accepted you will notify you about the types of aid for which you are eligible, usually through an award letter. Consider some of the following scholarship and grant options:

- Many postsecondary institutions use the *Federal Perkins Loan Program* to help students pay for their education. After five years of full-time work as a PA, the loan pays itself off through an annual cancellation and deferment process.[2] Two separate forms are required to apply: a Perkins promissory note and the FAFSA.
- The *National Health Service Corps* (NHSC) supports primary-care providers in underserved areas. Students can apply for this scholarship before school, or apply for a loan-repayment option on completion of training. The loan repayment is tax-free.[3] See Chapter 8 in this book for an "inside look" by a scholarship recipient about her experience.
- Applying for *private scholarships* is another excellent option. Spend time doing research from October through December because many deadlines for applications are January through April.

The best website to begin your research on private education loans is www.finaid.org/loans/privatestudentloans.phtml. It contains a comprehensive list of lenders and advice on how to research your best match for a lender.

The following databases are recommended to search for scholarships:

- www.collegeanswer.com/paying/scholarship_search/pay_scholar ship_search.jsp
- http://apps.collegeboard.com/cbsearch_ss/welcome.jsp
- www.fastweb.com/college-scholarships
- www.scholarships.com/
- www.collegenet.com/mach25/app
- www.nerdwallet.com/education/scholarships/index.php

The College Board also publishes a scholarship handbook that is very useful: http://store.collegeboard.com/sto/productdetail.do?Itemkey=009713

How Do You Know Whether the Scholarships You Find Are Legitimate?

These are a few things to be aware of when looking for scholarship opportunities:

1. Be weary of scams that ask you to send money with the application.
2. Check the status of the offering group on the Better Business Bureau (BBB) website to verify legitimacy.
3. Exclusivity (e.g., sign up for subscription, "like" us on Facebook) is questionable.
4. Lottery draws are not legitimate.
5. Check out Fastweb's warning signs for more information: www. fastweb.com/college-scholarships/articles/54-10-scam-warning-signs.[4]

Little Steps to Big Savings

1. *Set a budget, and live within your means.* "Buy what you absolutely *need*, and not what you *want*" is a motto to live by. Before you start school, take the time to evaluate your monthly expenses. Look at items such as your car insurance, cell phone plan, cable television plan, and subscriptions. Downgrade where possible, and cancel any unnecessary luxuries. Keep track of your expenses, and adjust accordingly.
2. *Consider alternatives.* You may not need to *own* each and every book on the recommended school list. Research the option of downloading e-books, buying used books, renting your textbooks, or checking the book out of the school library.
3. *Keep it local.* To save money on apartment furnishings and transportation costs, consider on-campus apartments that are fully furnished.
4. *Be smart about your money.* Sometimes a membership fee can lead to big savings. For example, consider getting an American Automobile Association (AAA) membership. It costs roughly $75 per year, and you receive discounts on travel, insurance, restaurants, shopping, tickets to attractions throughout the United States,

discounted automobile insurance, and free roadside assistance. *Take advantage of loyalty programs.* Sign up for shopper's discount cards at the places you shop the most.

5. *BYO.* Brew your own coffee in the morning and bring your own packed lunch instead of purchasing individual cups of coffee and eating out. You can save at least $10 a day, or $200 per month. Avoid vending machines by bringing your own drinks and snacks to school.

6. *Party at home.* Stay in with friends to cook or make cocktails rather than going out.

7. *Think big.* When the price per unit of everyday household items, such as toilet paper, shampoo, and soap, is cheaper, buy these items in bulk.

8. *Have a no-debt policy.* Avoid nonacademic debt, such as credit-card debt, automobile debt, and incurring fees because of bank over-drafts. If you use a credit card, do not spend more money than you actually have in the bank.

9. *Be true to yourself.* Do not spend time with "big spenders." Avoid "keeping up with the Joneses," and stay true to your budget.

10. *Read your labels.* Buy machine-washable clothes so that you can minimize the use of expensive dry-cleaning services.

COURSEWORK LOAD

PA school is not like undergraduate school. The volume of information you are required to know and the pace at which you must learn it are accelerated. You are expected to read, understand, and retain the material. Finding yourself in highly stressful and competitive situations is inevitable. Run your own race. Your neighbor may be a "gunner" or a "slacker," and comparing yourself with him or her is a waste of energy. Focus on your-self. It is important to remember to take PA school one day at a time, and study without getting overwhelmed.

Eight Tips for Success in the Classroom

1. *Start out right to stay in balance.* In the initial months of PA school, develop healthy habits, such as staying organized and allotting a

healthy amount of study time and an appropriate amount of time to relax and recover.

2. *Pick the right seat in class.* Choose to sit in a place where you will pay attention and not get distracted.

3. *Get help early.* The first time you don't understand something, go ask the professor during the break or after class. Seek tutoring resources at your institution to stay on top of the subject matter.

4. *Preview to prepare.* Go over the material that will be covered in class *prior* to the lecture in order to better absorb the material.

5. *Get enough sleep.* A rested brain absorbs more.

6. *Do not procrastinate.* Instead of studying right before the exam, review the daily notes taken at the end of each class day. Cramming is not an effective way to study because each exam covers too much material.

7. *Prioritize your studying.* First, study the material that you find is the most difficult. Save the easier topics for later.

8. *Take a break.* Have an outlet such as a sport, the gym, music, friends, or family. Avoid excessive amounts of alcohol as a way to wind down. Relax in a healthy way.

It is almost guaranteed that a PA student will have times of panic and frustration while in PA school. After some trial and error, I found it best to just complete one task at a time. It is important to budget your time with each task or assignment so you don't accidentally spend all of your time studying for just one class.

—Sarah Esther Hwang MPAP, PA-C

Put the effort in and do PA school right. The material you learn during your two to three years is all you get before that piece of paper that lets you go practice medicine. Do not regress to high school or college cramming techniques. Take the time to study every day. Please remember that you must understand and comprehend the material, not just learn it for the exam. That being said, create balance in your lifestyle, even if it is "chaotic balance." . . . Find an outlet, for me it was running, and it does not count if you're running while studying on the treadmill. . . . My friends and I created Sunday night dinners. We would rotate who hosted and would watch an episode of *Grey's Anatomy* after dinner.

—Jennifer Nowaczyk PA-C

Always maintain perspective. Instead of "I have to go to class," think, "I get to go to class." I know it sounds cheesy, but fake the enthusiasm. Haven't you heard of the motto, "Fake it till you make it"? Take a breath and picture yourself being awesome at whatever challenge that lies ahead. Say to yourself, "I am going to be the master of _____." Become your vision.

—Natasha Ohta PA-S

Just remember when you start to feel overwhelmed, you are not alone. We have all been there, and we got through it. If one class is really difficult for you, for example, dermatology, and you aren't interested in dermatology, let it go. In the end, when you pass the test, the initials after your name will still read PA-C. They will not say PA-C that got a B minus in dermatology. Your future employer and your future patients will not know the individual test grades in each class.

—Rebecca Isaacson PA-C

STUDY TECHNIQUES

Some people learn by seeing, some by doing, and others by hearing. For most, learning involves a combination of all of the above. Understanding how you absorb information is crucial. As obvious as it may seem, study techniques in PA school depend on the subject matter and an individual's personality. For classes that require a lot of reading, typing notes while reading may be most ideal. For rote memorization, note cards may be helpful. Writing out your own practice tests and quizzes is another useful technique. For the Objective Structured Clinical Examinations (OSCEs), working with a partner is valuable because you will be practicing physical examination techniques, such as using the ophthalmoscope or the otoscope, or checking reflexes. Microsoft OneNote worked very well for one student. It is a virtual notebook that allows for separate folders for each lecture. Notes from professors and images from the Internet can easily be added. It works especially well for visual topics such as dermatology and head, eyes, ears, nose, and throat (HEENT). Try a variety of study techniques at the beginning, and then stick with what works best for you. Study *smarter*, not *harder*. Turn off your cell phone, and avoid distractions while you are studying.

Group study sessions work well for some, but not for others. Working with fellow classmates can help with recall and integration of the material because you talk out loud and compare understandings. Classmates can lend a fresh perspective and help to solidify information in your memory. For some people, however, being with a group of people can be distracting. Idle chatter and storytelling can easily dilute the productivity of a study session if the group is not disciplined. Some students like this distraction because it makes studying more bearable. For others, this environment requires tolerance and patience to avoid frustration. Choose your group study partners wisely. A group is most effective when all the members prepare the material before meeting with each other.

Helpful Tips

1. *Find your "best" study spot.* Choose a place that allows you to maximize productivity, such as a quiet library, a coffee shop, or your home. Be careful when studying at home because there are many distractions, such as the television, the refrigerator, and your bed. Pick an environment that is most conducive to effective studying.

2. *Block out the noise.* Use earplugs or, better yet, purchase noise-canceling headphones so that you can study virtually anywhere with limited distractions.

3. *Pick the right partner.* If having a study partner works for you, find one who is dependable, disciplined, and encouraging. It is important to find a partner who is focused on the task at hand and who is as committed as you are. He or she must be reliable enough to show up on time when you arrange sessions. You will be wasting your time if your partner is there to talk socially or is ill-prepared.

4. *Organize your notes.* Rewrite notes to compile an organized packet for future studying. This can be very time-consuming, but if time allows, it will help you to retain the information.

5. *Know before you go.* Do not move forward in studying the next subject area until you fully understand the core concept in front of you. There is a slim chance that you will go back to relearn that section.

6. *Make it visual.* Draw charts and use colors to assist with visual recall. For human anatomy, redraw the book diagram and then make an attempt to redraw the image from memory.

7. *Play it back.* Read a summarized version of your own notes into a dictation tape, and listen while driving or exercising.

8. *Check your recall.* Quiz yourself regularly to retain information.

9. *Talk the talk.* Carpool or eat lunch with another student in order to talk the notes out loud.

10. *Discover.* The key is to find what works best for you in the PA program protocol. What worked for you as an undergraduate student may not work for you as a graduate student. Be flexible and open to other ideas.

TIME MANAGEMENT SKILLS

Time management is key in an accelerated one-year didactic program. PA school may be the most difficult academic challenge you have ever faced, and it requires discipline. Remaining organized is crucial. In order to stay on top of the daily demands of the program, one PA student dedicated a three-hour block each Sunday night to take care of the weekday preparation. She would grocery shop, prepare five lunches, and do laundry to feel prepared and less distracted for the week.

During each week of the first didactic year of PA school, an average PA student will typically spend

- 35 to 40 hours in class
- 20 to 40 hours studying
- 40 to 55 hours sleeping
- 0 to 10 hours exercising
- 7 to 15 hours relaxing with family and friends
- 1 to 3 hours commuting

Once you find an allocation of time that works for you, stick with what works.

SUPPORT SYSTEM

The PA program will test you mentally and emotionally, so it is important to have a good support system. Classmates can empathize with what you are going through. It is also important to make time for your friends and family, even if it is only a few minutes daily on the phone to tell them how much they mean to you. Some PA programs have a separate orientation for their students' family members. If such an orientation is offered, I encourage you to have them attend so that they can better understand the demands of your schooling and offer you appropriate support. Some schools offer a big-brother/big-sister program. If this is an option, take part in it. Seek out a PA mentor.

The didactic portion of PA school requires focus, discipline, and the understanding that this short-course program has an end in sight. Stay positive, and remember, all PAs had to experience a similar didactic year, and they persevered. This training is necessary to the build the foundation of your medical knowledge. You will see in Chapter 4 that the clinical portion of PA school is hands-on and, therefore, much more appealing. Instead of being hunched over a book, you will be standing over a human body in the operating room (OR). Or instead of reading words on a page about a specific disease, such as systemic lupus erythematous (SLE), you will experience it firsthand. Instead of reviewing the signs and symptoms of the disease through a textbook, you will talk to patients and hear their systemic complaints, observe the malar butterfly rash, and get a firsthand look at the lab results of anemia, thrombocytopenia, and protein spilled in the urine. Seeing things "live" in the second year fills in all the question marks you had in the first year, and everything comes together. The point is—study smart in your first year so that you can build your medical knowledge and apply what you have learned during your clinical year of PA school.

References

1. Free Application for Federal Student Aid (FAFSA), 2012; available at: www.fafsa.ed.gov.

2. U.S. Department of Education, Federal Perkins Loan Program, 2012; available at: www2.ed.gov/programs/fpl/index.html.

3. U.S. Department of Health and Human Services, National Health Service Corps, 2012; http://nhsc.hrsa.gov/.

4. Zubia, A. Financial Aid Counselor, Western University of Health Sciences.

[CHAPTER 4]

Physician Assistant Student Life

INTRODUCTION

As a student, you have high expectations for hands-on learning, performing procedures, and building confidence in your clinical skills during rotations.[1] Your preceptor, otherwise known as your supervising physician, will be more enthusiastic about teaching you if you are prepared. As you plan your clinical year, take advantage of as many student rotational opportunities as possible. Use this time to add depth and breadth to your skill set.

> I went to New York for a month to experience a new environment in a rural hospital as the only student in the emergency department (ED). This opportunity allowed for one-on-one learning, and I was able to gain quality experience in suturing, incision and drainage procedures, foreign-body removals, and intubating.

If your school allows, take a trip to a rural location or do an international rotation to broaden your medical knowledge and cultural experiences. In most cases, a rotation is what *you* make of it.[1] During a hospital or clinic rotation, be present in activities your preceptor invites you to, such as medical staff meetings, grand rounds, or evening continuing medical education (CME) programs.[1] This will provide you with insight and an enhanced perspective to the real world of clinical practice.

Rotations provide you with the opportunity to literally step into the lives of complete strangers and work with them side by side for 4 to 6 weeks at a time. You will be challenged with learning new names and faces, managing interpersonal dynamics, gaining exposure to a variety of medical conditions and resulting procedures, and adjusting to the practice style of your supervising physician. For the first time, you may be caring for patients of different socioeconomic classes, such as a homeless intravenous drug abuser with multiple medical problems. At times, you may feel overwhelmed, but the experience ultimately will prove to be invaluable. This chapter provides preparation guidelines and practical tips for your clinical rotations. It also includes six "day in the life of a physician assistant student" excerpts from students writing about their experience in physician assistant (PA) school.

Clinical Rotations

General Preparation

Make sure that your immunizations are up to date. Influenza and H1N1 vaccinations are required in many hospitals and clinics. Carry proof of your hepatitis, varicella, and rubella titers and negative purified protein derivative (PPD) records. Know your school's policy for the exposure-control plan for blood-borne and airborne pathogens and who to contact if an exposure should occur. Hospital sites should fit your face for a tuberculosis (TB) mask because a proper fit is required to prevent airborne exposure. Research the community in which you will be working, and check online to search the U.S. Census Bureau State and County Quick Facts.[1] Try to learn pertinent information about your supervising physician or PA before you meet. Research where he or she went to school and whether he or she has any published works. Watch videos online of some of the procedures you may be doing.

Academic Preparation

Have your "SOAP note" methodology memorized.[1] The note, incorporating *subjective* and *objective* information and the *assessment* and *plan*, is adaptable for each subspecialty or rotation. The *subjective* component is the patient's reason for seeking medical care, which includes the *chief complaint* in the patient's own words and the history of present illness (HPI) in narrative form. The *objective* component includes vital signs, physical examination, and laboratory results or diagnostic tests. The *assessment* is the medical diagnosis pertaining to the chief complaint derived from a list of possible diagnoses, referred to as *differential diagnoses*. The *plan* includes treatment, instruction, and recommendations for follow-up.

Student Etiquette

First impressions are important. Your preceptor and coworkers for the next month will form an opinion about you based on your appearance, clothing, body language, and demeanor. This first encounter is nearly impossible to undo and sets the tone for the relationship.[1] Be calm and confident, stand with good posture, smile, make eye contact, and greet people with a firm handshake.[2] Introduce yourself to the secretary and all other medical staff associated with your supervising physician. These staff members are tremendous assets who can provide you with valuable assistance as you adjust to each new rotation. Give the office manager your business card and contact information in case there are last-minute schedule changes. Ask about dress code, student workspace, reference materials, hours of operation, and additional learning opportunities.[1]

Initially, you may feel completely disoriented. Do not expect to know all the answers. Even though you may feel fearful when asked, "Do you want to do this procedure?" Say, "Yes!" You are there to learn, and there is a first time for everything. If you are asked something that you do not know, say, "I don't know, but I will look it up and get back to you." And *do* get back to the person in a timely manner. Some rotations will "hand hold" by giving you an orientation and will let you completely shadow on the first day or even the first week. Other rotations will "throw you straight to the lions" and will expect you to round on patients independently and write notes on the first day. Since your supervising physician changes every 4 to 6 weeks, this pattern may alternate, and it may be difficult to adjust to. Never assume your role. Ask your preceptor what his or her expectations are, how he or she wants the case presentations formatted, and his or her preferred method of giving you feedback. Physician assistant schools usually have objectives for each rotation. Review these in conjunction with the supervising physician, and ask for a formal midterm evaluation. Refer to the "Physician Assistant Competencies" in Chapter 2, and work toward meeting those expectations.[1]

Know your place as a student. You are representing your school as well as the PA profession. Remember that you are stepping into a short-term role in an established medical practice. This is your preceptor's workplace and livelihood, and for you, this is a brief learning experience. The patients you see are his or her patients. Be receptive to learning, even if it is learning the hard way or being reprimanded. Be open to constructive criticism. Never say, "How am I doing?" Instead, ask for 5 minutes to sit down and address a topic you want to talk about.[1] Request honest feedback, and act on those recommendations.

> At the end of one long 16-hour day, my supervising physician questioned my actions and then scolded me. I cried in front of him. Never cry! For the rest of the rotation, and in front of other people, he would comment, "Are you okay? Am I going to make you cry today?"

Arrive early every day. It's better to be an hour early than 5 minutes late. Consider each rotation as if it were a month-long interview for a potential job. Dress professionally. Wear minimal jewelry and fragrance, cover exposed tattoos, and do not chew gum. For men, appear neatly groomed with a clean-shaven face, short hair, and trimmed fingernails. For women, avoid bringing a purse. There is not always a convenient place to store it, which means that you may need to place it in an unsafe or unclean environment. Instead, put any necessities in your lab coat pockets. Women also should avoid wearing heels because you never know how much walking or standing will be required of you. Dress appropriately for any scenario.

> On my obstetrics rotation, I wore heels and brought a purse on my first day. For this rotation I was told I would be in clinic, but we got called immediately to the hospital for a delivery. I walked into the Labor and Delivery Department and had to put scrub booties on over heels, which is a safety hazard, with potential to slip. The nurses rolled their eyes at me, and I heard indiscriminate whispering when I asked where to put my purse.

Professional Etiquette

The PA student-to-patient relationship is important for both parties. Practice good bedside manners to establish excellent rapport with your patients. When walking into a patient room, always introduce yourself as a PA student, and shake hands with the patient. Maintain eye contact with the patient while taking a history. Do not share personal stories about yourself, even if they seem pertinent to the patient's complaint. When performing an examination, always explain what you are doing. While listening to the lungs, place the stethoscope on the patient's bare skin, never over clothing. And most important, think before you speak.

> On my obstetrics rotation, it was common to perform a well-woman exam on patients. After completing one woman's pelvic and breast examination, I said, "Everything looked good." I was corrected by my attending physician to *never say that* and to instead say, "Your exam was normal."

Read and adhere to the Health Insurance Portability and Accountability Act (HIPAA) guidelines. For example, taking pictures of a patient's examination findings is a HIPAA violation unless the photo is being placed in their medical record or unless you have signed consent.[1]

Before you leave a rotation, speak with the office manager for the best mailing address, and get business cards for the correct spelling of all support staff. Send a hand-written thank-you note within a week of completing the rotation.

Inevitably, you will make mistakes, and hopefully, you learn from them. "Mistakes are painful when they happen, but years later, a collection of mistakes is what is called experience."[3] Make the very most out of your clinical rotations. Work hard to develop good habits while learning medicine. This is the foundational year for your knowledge and physical examination skills. Think of your rotational year as the start of your professional career rather than a continuation of your education.

Resources

1. Lord, Cynthia B., MHS, PA-C. "Surviving Clinical Rotations Lecture," Quinnipiac University, Physician Assistant Program, AAPA Toronto Conference, May 2012.

2. Mind Tools. "Essential Skills for an Excellent Career, Making a Great First Impression, Getting Off to a Good Start," 2012. Available at: www.mindtools.com/CommSkll/FirstImpressions.htm.

3. Quote by Denis Waitly. Available at: http://www.searchquotes.com/Denis_Waitley/Mistakes/quotes/

A DAY IN THE LIFE: DIDACTIC PA YEAR

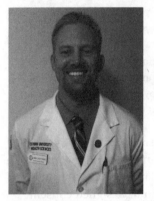

Daniel Hestehauge, PA-S

It is the third week of PA school, and I am already feeling overwhelmed. I've spent almost my entire weekend studying, except for a few hours going out to dinner with my wife. Physician assistant school is nothing like my undergrad days. Back then, I could finish my homework in a matter of minutes and study for exams the night before. Now I read for hours, review notes nonstop, and keep my bloodstream flowing with caffeine. Nine classes in one semester? Is this even possible? Let's not forget about the three exams, two quizzes, and physical assessment checklist I have coming up this week. This is quickly becoming the most challenging experience of my life.

And so, another Monday begins . . .

6:00 a.m.

My alarm goes off, I take a deep breath, and I mentally prepare myself for the day. By waking up early, I can get an extra 3 hours of studying in before class.

7:15 a.m.

I arrive at the school library carrying a backpack filled with medical books, a laptop bag across one shoulder, and my lunch bag over the other. My friends and I meet together in a study room of the library every morning. Working in small groups (larger groups can become distracting) has made me realize that everyone brings a different way of understanding the material to the table, and when you're able to talk through the material with others, it makes it that much easier to learn.

10:00 a.m.

The first class of the day is physical assessment. It is one of my favorites. One hour is dedicated to hands-on learning. Our professors demonstrate physical examination techniques, and we practice in small groups. Today we are focusing on cardiology physical examination techniques; skills will give me clues to a potentially life-threatening heart condition that one day may save someone's life.

The second hour is dedicated to lecture. Cases are presented, and pictures of pertinent physical examination findings are shown. Figuring out your best way to absorb the material is critical. I started the school year taking notes on my computer along with just about everyone else in my class, but I realized that I was spending more time typing things that were already given to me in a handout instead of actually listening to the professor. So I started printing every handout I was given before class and writing additional notes by hand. I felt more engaged in the lectures, and I was absorbing the material much more effectively. As you can imagine, the notes and paper piled up very quickly, so I bought a binder with dividers for every class and organized them accordingly. When it came time to studying for the exam, I had everything I needed in one place, and my eyes were relieved that they didn't have to stare at a computer screen all day.

12:00 p.m.

Class has just ended, and word has spread quickly that our grades from our exam last week have been put into our lockers, so during our lunch break, we all took off running. The results were from our first adult medicine exam of the year. I opened my locker and pulled out the results. Eighty-four percent. I passed! What an amazing feeling it is to know that my hard work paid off. After all my doubts, it was a rewarding feeling that makes me feel like, "You can do this!"

My classmate Joey, on the other hand, wasn't so happy. He had worked seemingly just as hard as everyone else and had failed his exam. After going to test review, he realized that he had been studying wrong. Joey was used to memorizing and seeing questions as only having one answer. Unfortunately, PA school is more about understanding than memorizing. Similarly, practicing medicine is about applying concepts and recognizing the most likely correct answer rather than the only correct answer. Joey not only went to test review but was then plugged into our school's tutoring program.

1:00 p.m.

The second class for the day is adult medicine. This is the core of our didactic training. Here we learn about some of the most important and common disease states and conditions that we will see in practice. This class is broken up into nine core units that take approximately 1 month each. The units include Head, Ears, Eyes, Nose, and Throat (HEENT); Pulmonary; Cardiology; Dermatology; Gastroenterology; Orthopedics; Neurology; Hematology; and Infectious Disease. We learn the major disease states of each unit and are expected to know the pathophysiology, presentation, labs, diagnostic studies, and treatments for each disease state. When tested on this material, the questions are often written in a case-presentation format describing a patient's symptoms or lab results, and the answer may require you to know both the diagnosis and treatment to get the answer correct.

Most of our time is spent studying for this class. A small group of us has decided to divide out the unit objectives to help see the material in different ways. For every unit, we set a deadline for the work to be completed and posted online so that we all have ample time to look it over and study from it before the exam. It's an excellent way to see the reading in a different format and make sure that we have met all the objectives for that topic. It also can be a nice review after we have finished our own reading and helps to condense the reading into more manageable chunks by highlighting key points. It is important to remember, however, not to rely on other people's work. We should always do the assigned reading on our own—and probably more than once.

3:30 p.m.

After adult medicine, we get a short break until we have to meet in the laboratory for clinical skills. Today we are learning how to do blood draws. Most of my classmates have experience doing blood draws. In this brief workshop, we get a demonstration of the instruments and the technique used for introducing the needle into a vein. It seemed simple enough, but I quickly learned it was more challenging than I had thought. My partner drew my blood first because she was a nurse before starting PA school, and it could not have gone any smoother. Then it was my turn. My hands start sweating uncontrollably. I find the vein and prepare the site. I pick up the syringe and pull off the cap to the needle. As I start to bring the needle closer to my partner's arm, my hands start to shake. After a few moments and deep breaths, I finally completed the task. I was surprised at how a simple procedure such as a blood draw took so much skill and precision.

5:15 p.m.

After our skills lab, I realized that the next time I would be doing a blood draw would be on a real patient. We congratulated each other on another successful day and left for home.

7:00 p.m.

After a nice dinner with my wife, it's time to study again. Most weeknights I can get 3 to 6 hours of studying done. Even when I don't have an exam or quiz the next day, I still take the time to read. I've learned that time management is one of the most important survival skills of PA school. If you wait until the last minute for everything, you will not do well. Studying a little at a time keeps your mind sharp and makes learning easier. I always try to keep my eye on the goal and remind myself why I am doing this.

A DAY IN THE LIFE: PA STUDENT ROTATIONS

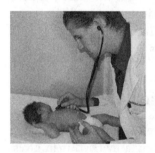

Daniel McConnell, Jr., MS, PA-S

A day in the life of a PA student (PA-S) can be likened to one's freshman year of high school. No matter where you go (hospital, clinic, or operating room), you will be the low man or woman on the totem pole. To accentuate this scene, you'll also be the only one wearing your short white coat, whereas the seasoned PAs and physicians wear longer white coats. Your title will be "The Student" for the next year because physicians, nurses, and medical assistants will persistently introduce you to their comrades as such. Sounds intimidating; however, just like high school, it is what you make of it. Never in life will you have the opportunity to meet as many healthcare professionals or learn without the full responsibility of your own license weighing solely on your shoulders.

Instead of a classic day in the life of a PA student, I gave a portion of my day in the following rotations: orthopedic surgery, obstetrics, general surgery, and emergency medicine.

8 a.m.: Orthopedic Surgery Center

"Do you know how to scrub?" my preceptor asks. "Absolutely," I say, sounding like an overzealous student. I was fully aware that every physician I'd worked for up to this point had very different definitions of scrubbing in (some were meticulous, others weren't). "Good, you're first assist. We're doing an anterior cruciate ligament (ACL) repair on a 16-year-old soccer player."

Swinging open the door to operating room B, I see a thin young-looking leg being prepped by the surgical nurse and tech. The surgeon accounts for all the necessary tools he will use to craft the new ACL, and I stand quietly and participate when asked. He makes his final anatomic marks on the patient's left thigh and lower leg and begins to question me on each site. I fare well but am completely blank when asked, "Which tendons will be *autografts* for this patient?" Utter silence occurs for the better part of 15 seconds as I hope for him to answer, but he doesn't. Minutes later, he holds both tendons in his hand as if they are fish on a line and proudly exclaims, "The semitendinosus and the gracilis." I imagine he is smiling, but I can only see his eyes because of his surgical mask.

We walk over to a table in the corner of the room and begin to shape, fold, and braid the graft to provide appropriate strength and size. The surgeon gives approval and walks back to the patient to thread the graft through the proximal tibia and distal femur, fixating both ends with screws. From open to close, the entire operation is just over an hour.

11:15 a.m.: Women's Health Clinic

There aren't many things that horrify male PA students as much as anticipating their ob-gyn rotation. I must say that being a married man gives me a head start, but not by much. As I walk into the women's health clinic located inside the hospital, I realize that there is an excess of estrogen and a deficiency of testosterone. Most of the physicians, medical staff, and students are female. The population is also predominately Spanish-speaking.

"Habla ingles o Espanol?" I ask my first patient. "No hablo ingles, solamente espanol," she claims. "Me llamo es Daniel, soy estudiante de medicinas. Que problemas ahora?" I stumble steadily through my questions and gather what information I can. I realize that this young Hispanic woman is here for her first prenatal visit, and she is unsure how far along she is. She has recently come to the United States from Mexico with her husband and two children. She is uncertain about her last menstrual period and has not had an ultrasound. I examine her for fetal heart tones and fundal height: 140–150 beats/min and 20 cm. I approach my attending physician and let her know about the circumstances, and she asks me what I would like to do. "I think she needs an ultrasound to determine her expected date of delivery," I said. She agrees and performs the ultrasound as I observe and learn that the baby is measuring 18 weeks and 5 days.

As any good student does, I glance at my cheat sheet to see what this patient needs today. I walk back into the patient's room with the interpreter because the details of this conversation exceed my Spanish-language abilities. I teach her about alpha-fetoprotein (AFP) testing for neural tube defects, quickening (fetal movements), Braxton-Hicks contractions, and finally, diet and exercise recommendations. I ask her, "Entiende?" And she replies, "Si doctor, gracias." I know I should correct her about my title being a PA student, but under pressure, I am not sure how. So, in closing, I say, "No problema, Senora, le ver en cuatro semanas."

1:45 p.m.: General Surgery

I find myself scrubbing in once again for an appendectomy. Most general surgery rotations are filled with "appy's and chole's," as was mine. I figure that this one will take less than an hour because the patient is a young man with the typical presentation of appendicitis. He has a 2-day history of fever, anorexia, vomiting, and right lower quadrant abdominal pain that started out periumbilically. Classic, right?

My preceptor does arthroscopic surgeries 99 percent of the time, and the same was true today. My job as his first assistant is to hold the camera steady so that he can see both his tools while in the peritoneal space. Sounds easy, but it's not. Your right is left, and your down is up. We could not find the appendix! While I'm on the camera, he's sifting through the small and large intestine, and nothing; then we would switch, still nothing.

After 30 minutes of searching for the hidden treasure otherwise known as the "pirate's appy," we stare at each other in disbelief. He finally says, "let's open him up," and seconds later he makes a 10-cm incision in the right lower quadrant medial to the anteriosuperior iliac spine (ASIS).

Together, we find a *retroperitoneal* appendix and notice that it's enlarged, purple, and ruptured. "Bag it," my preceptor says, as he dilutes the peritoneal space and places the Jackson-Pratt (JP) drain. I sew and he staples to close. Relief settles in the operating room (OR). I learn very early in my student career that very few things go according to plan, especially when they're considered "classic."

3:25 p.m.: Emergency Department

"Scientist first, humanist second," a great veteran PA once told me as he explained what my role would be in the medical field. Fairly easy to have them flow from the mouth, yet these words offer an internal struggle if chosen to live by.

As I walk the halls of the Emergency Department, I glance down to room 49's medical record. A 3-year-old boy complains of right wrist and arm pain for the last 2 hours. I enter the room and listen to the father tell me, quite expressionless, that his son was at a day-care center and ran into a wall after being chased. I step out of the room and walk with my preceptor to review the boy's x-rays. The results are alarming because the boy suffers from a severely displaced distal radius and ulnar fracture inconsistent with the mechanism (at least to me). Science takes a backseat, and I incline to observe the situation as an abusive one.

"We should probably get social services involved," I plead. Indifferent, my preceptor has two other physicians also check in on the little guy. The results: Reduce it, splint him up, and refer to ortho. I watch the father and his 3-year-old walk out of the ED, the boy quietly says, "Thank you." The father says nothing. No one will ever really know the truth behind the injury. Right or wrong, I hang my hat on the fact three other sets of eyes were laid on the situation, and the decision was made with all opinions considered.

With clinical rotations complete, the "S" in PA-S now stands for survivor because I have finished my career as a student and am now facing the world of responsibilities. It is a year I will never forget. I look forward to the next chapter, and I am very thankful for all my experiences.

A DAY IN THE LIFE: GENERAL SURGERY PA STUDENT ROTATION

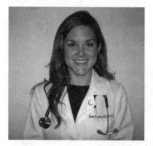

Sarah Broome, MS, PA-C

As a child, I never believed that I would pursue a career in medicine; however, I would play doctor to my pets and siblings by cleaning their wounds with antiseptic and gently applying a Band-Aid. All my "patients" were resigned to my incessant need to deliver medical care at such a young age. No one in my family had pursued a career in medicine. I had no idea what "a day in the life" of a PA would be like until my first PA student rotation in general surgery. It has come to be one of the most fulfilling and spiritually uplifting weeks of my life. For the sake of following a patient's case to completion, I combined the events that occurred over a week timespan into this story. This week will always be a reminder of why I made the best decision to pursue a career as a PA.

7:18 a.m.: Rounding

Sleepily, I pull into the parking lot of one of the three hospitals we performed surgeries at throughout the day. The day starts with rounding. I know it's after 7 a.m., but I am tired, exhausted actually. We had an emergency appendectomy last night on an 8-year-old girl that lasted until 2 a.m. My "cowboy" attending surgeon (the name I have quietly assigned him) never stops, requires little sleep, and rarely eats. It appears that he lives purely on adrenaline and Diet Coke. We go from case to case, racing from hospital to hospital, and then to his community clinic every day, all day. We have been putting in 12- to 14-hour days and returning for emergent surgeries that end after midnight for the last 2 weeks. As my first rotation of my clinical year, I am struggling to keep up with this intense pace!

I enter the hospital, print my list of patients, and shuffle down the first floor headed toward my first patient. Because I am new to my clinical year, my lab coat is loaded with reference books, instruments, gauze packs, adhesive tape, rulers, and a granola bar in the case that lunch doesn't happen again. My cell rings with my attending surgeon's number.

I answer, and he quickly says to do an H&P (a history and physical write-up) on a new patient who was admitted this morning for nonspecific rectal bleeding. I add her to my list of 21 patients. It's going to be another long day.

8:30 a.m.: New Admits

After rounding on a few other patients, I enter the new admit's room. She is a pleasant 65-year-old Hispanic woman lying on her hospital bed. I begin by introducing myself as a PA student working with the general surgeon. She looks puzzled and laughs. I immediately learn that she only speaks Spanish, and I begin again. My undergraduate degree in Spanish literature is coming in handy, and I am thankful for the practice. I learn that she had noticed significant bleeding after a bowel movement for the past few weeks. She is anemic, and I notice her pale complexion. She has not been to a doctor since her last child was born 35 years ago, takes no medication, has no past medical or surgical history. In school, I am conditioned to assume cancer in an elderly person with unexplained bleeding until proven otherwise, but I still hate to consider it. I ask "¿Alguien en tu familia ha tenido cancer?" She shakes her head in no. I finish with my questions, and before I leave, she takes my hand and thanks me, "Gracias, Momi."

Probably just a hemorrhoid, I think. I hope. The surgeon recommends a colonoscopy and blood work.

On to the next patient . . .

9:18 a.m.: Challenges and Comfort

The most challenging patient we currently have on our service and a long-time resident of the hospital is ready and waiting with her daily rant. She immediately starts yelling, "When am I going to get outta here? I am ready to go home, I've got to get out of here!!" She is a morbidly obese woman with an extensive medical history including chronic obstructive pulmonary disease (COPD), hypothyroidism, diabetes, chronic kidney disease stage 3, hypertension, hypercholesterolemia, and newly diagnosed colon cancer. The complexity of her comorbid conditions is overwhelming, especially to the new second-year PA student. She is a kind woman at heart who explains that she became overwhelmed by some obstacles in her personal life that ultimately lead to the degradation of her health. She admits that she is anxious to return home to help her only daughter with her schoolwork.

I gently examen her healing extensive abdominal incision from a 6-hour complicated open colon resection 3 days prior. As I head for the doorway, I reassure her that we are trying to help her, and as I leave, she appears calm again and is thanking me. She is teaching me one of my most important instruments as a future provider—compassion. She reminds me that I have the ability to provide great comfort to my patients.

10:05 a.m.: Let's Hurry Up to Wait

New to the clinical world, I work at about the speed of a tortoise while rounding and writing SOAP (*s*ubjective, *o*bjective, *a*ssessment, and *p*lan) notes. My SOAP notes look like small novels. The other seasoned PAs, nurse practitioners (NPs), and physicians scribble a few lines and numbers with a quick signature and are on their way.

I get the text, "Surgery at 10:15 at the other hospital." I'll have to come back to finish rounding on the remaining patients later.

I walk quickly into the OR corridor and find my surgeon. He is wrapped in a warm postoperative room blanket and is reviewing our patient list on the computer because the surgery is delayed. In surgery, I have learned that it is best to be silent and, when prompted, to give short, relevant reports on your patients. His stern and challenging questions regarding our patients' conditions and plans require considerable mental effort and immediate rebound from the occasional humility and embarrassment of a wrong answer. Our relationship involves understood silence, my questions and his one-word answers, his questions and my fear-filled responses, and some occasional teasing. He is an excellent teacher who gives his students the feeling of having great responsibility while he quietly watches over you 100 percent.

We get into the OR, scrubbed and ready. With only 2 weeks in surgery, the high volume of procedures I have done gives me confidence in this routine. I am still afraid of the scrub nurse, whose motto is, "Don't touch anything blue!" As a new student, you walk into the OR looking like you are able to perform some complicated martial arts moves through a laser-filled obstacle course; sterile hands above elbows while dodging the fast-paced nurses and techs prepping the patient.

The surgery goes well—just another laparoscopic appendectomy. The surgeon trusts me to close the incision under his close supervision. He corrects my technique initially and then allows me to finish. I think I must be improving. I celebrate with a silent internal cheer. Approval is the greatest gift for any student.

I thank the team and exit the OR. I change into new scrubs and return to rounding on patients.

1:45 p.m.: Hospital Food

Iceberg lettuce, Saltine cracker packets, and cold cuts are the options for my 5-minute lunch break. I give a quick hello to a fellow classmate on her seemingly mellow cardiology rotation. She gets a whole hour to eat! The luxury, I think enviously, as I drive back to the first hospital to finish rounding.

2:15 p.m. (2 Days Later): Bad News

As I near the hospital entrance, I see two women sitting on the curb outside. One looks familiar, but I don't immediately place her. She stands up as I walk by, and she approaches me and says, "It's cancer," and she bursts into tears. I scramble to mentally place this woman. Then it comes to me—the sweet elderly Hispanic woman with the rectal bleeding. Her colonoscopy biopsy was positive for malignancy. My heart sinks. I find that my biggest challenge in this career is not letting my emotions get the best of me. My heart silently breaks for my patients and their families. I call my surgeon, and he tells me that he is already aware of the results. He instructs me to gather the family and meet him in the patient's room.

This is something they teach you in PA school practice scenarios, but there is no way to be truly prepared for your first real experience. You cannot prepare yourself for the patient's shock and grief as you deliver sad news and witness the emotion from the family. You hold the worst secret, and once you tell it, you hope that you can provide comfort and solace with a treatment plan.

The family meeting begins, and before anyone speaks, the family begins to cry. The woman does not. Instead, she fixates on the leather necklace around the surgeon's neck, a cross. She quickly reaches down the neck of her hospital gown and pulls out the same necklace. The stoic surgeon softens, and she grabs his hands. She places his hands onto her forehead, holding them there while praying. She is repeating that she isn't ready to go to the Lord yet and that this special doctor will help to save her. It's powerful, spiritual, and emotional. The surgeon's eyes fill with tears. This experience lasts 5 minutes. The surgeon and I leave together, and as we walk down the hallway, I notice that he has softened. His heart breaks also for his patients.

3 p.m. (2 days later): A Little Divine Intervention

We've looked at the imaging and explained the risks and benefits. The patient is ready—ready for surgery to resect the cancerous section of her colon. However, given the location of the cancer and other incidental findings on her computed tomographic (CT) scan, the surgeon will also have to perform a complete hysterectomy, appendectomy, and cholecystectomy. It is estimated to be a 4-hour surgery. In our earlier preoperative visit, the patient explained to me that she had a vision that Jesus and the Virgin Mary would also be present in the room this afternoon watching over her and guiding the surgical team. We are all praying for some divine intervention on this case.

I don't usually go into the OR when the patient is still conscious because it is usually quite busy, and I like to stay out of the way. This time I go in early to talk with her. She is comforted by my presence and responding, "Ok, Momi," just before she drifts under sedation. Time to get scrubbed.

The surgeon works carefully and efficiently. A fellow PA student joins us with the assistant surgeon. The two long-time partners work methodically, locating the appropriate regions and carefully cutting, clamping, removing, and suturing. My classmate and I hold instruments and assist occasionally, shifting our weight from one leg to the other during the long hours of the surgery. We watch in admiration of our teachers. Lastly, they complete an *anastomosis* with the remaining colon in order to prevent her from having a colostomy bag indefinitely. It is successful. My internal cheering is going wild. It's funny what you celebrate in medicine. We celebrate when you leave your patient in the most whole and most healed state, allowing her or him the most independence and integrity possible.

8 p.m.: Healing

The patient is quietly sleeping in the intensive-care unit (ICU), her body attempting to start the healing process after being significantly altered just hours ago. We hope for the best but understand some things are out of our control. I am hoping that this will turn out to be a miracle.

This day was a compilation of a week, as I stated in the introduction. A few days after the surgery, we learned that we were successful in removing the cancerous part of the colon, and this patient recovered well. The team of doctors decided that she was able to return home 1 week postoperatively without chemotherapy or radiation. She was discharged on my last day of my surgery rotation. I saved her for last during rounding because I wanted to take a little extra time to say goodbye. She hugged me and thanked me repetitively. She said she would pray for success and health in my life. She is a patient I will never forget. I gave one more quick wave goodbye as I left her room, and she whispered in English, "I love you, Momi."

This experience, filled with a wide range of emotions and challenges, tested my attitude and strength and will forever shape my clinical perspective. This rotation is a testament to what drew me to this career—a profession centered on providing compassion for others, sharing in spirituality, and exemplifying your steadfast daily commitment to provide the best care possible for your patients.

A DAY IN THE LIFE: GENERAL SURGERY PA STUDENT ROTATION

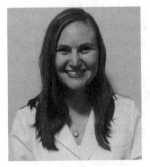

Casey Lorraine McCollum, PA-C

In the darkness, I arrive at Redlands Community Hospital to report for my first day as a general surgery physician assistant student (PA-S). My attending surgeon asked me to arrive at 7:15 a.m. Due to nerves and the fear of traffic making me late, I arrive at 6 a.m. To make the time pass, I watch online videos on my phone of the surgeries for the day.

7 a.m.

As the sun rises over the eastward mountains, I step into the five-story hospital building. The main entrance is nicely decorated with potted plants and wall murals, and luckily, the information desk is conveniently located, so I asked for further directions. A friendly hospital worker at the surgery entrance desk asks for my name, reviews my badge, makes a phone call, and allows me into the highly secured employee locker room. A whiteboard is hung in front of the surgical unit listing all the surgeons' names, the surgery being done, and which OR they will use. This guides me in the right direction.

7:15 a.m.

I change into OR scrubs, surgical booties, and a surgical hat as I tuck my new dress clothes away in a dusty locker. The locker room door leads me to the preoperation (OP) area, where I shake hands with the first patient of the day, a 60-year-old woman needing surgery to remove her parathyroid, the hormone-secreting gland next to the thyroid that regulates calcium in the body. She asks me if while we're in the OR we could also perform a nip and tuck. I smile at her, "I'm just the student, but I like your enthusiasm." At her bedside, I review the chart and flip through the pages to find something relevant to today's surgery. Just then my preceptor surgeon greets me and introduces me to his PA, Chris. I then become Chris's shadow. He makes me feel welcome by giving me a minitour of the OR. He checks my hand size and decides that I would wear a size 6.5 surgical glove.

7:30 a.m.

After much anticipation, it's finally time for my first OR experience. As sweat beads off my back, Chris demonstrates how to scrub in. Because the face mask and eyewear are not sterile, I put these on first before placing my hands under the running water. A sponge is provided, and Chris shows me how to properly clean my fingernails. I scrub and then rinse my arms, allowing the water to drip beyond my elbows while keeping my fingers upward.

Following the others, I back into the OR door holding my arms up. Everything looks blue. The sterile field has been prepped, and the surgery is about to begin. The OR nurse hands me a sterile towel and shows me how to dry my hands. She then opens my gown for me, and I put my arms through with my fingers barely poking through the cuffs. I spin around and tie my gown shut and then put the gloves on. I have passed the first test—not breaking the sterile field while gowning. Rules in the OR are steadfast. If you allow your hands to go above your nipples or below your navel while gowned and gloved, you must leave the OR and start over. There is no room for error because the rules of sterility are designed for the safety of the patient. I stand next to my preceptor for the duration of the surgery and keep my hands in proper position. It is exciting to closely observe the carotid vein and artery and watch skilled hands successfully remove the parathyroid adenoma.

9:30 a.m.

After the first surgery, I follow my preceptor into the recovery room and watch him write postoperative orders. I pay close attention and take notes because he warns me that this will be my job next week.

The next scheduled surgery is a laparoscopic cholecystectomy, the surgical removal of the gallbladder with a laparoscope. This is one of the most common surgeries general surgeons perform, and roughly 1 million patients undergo gallbladder removal every year. Because I know this will be a surgery that we perform daily on this rotation, I take mental notes of each step. First, antiseptic solution is spread across the belly, and three small incisions are nicked in the skin for the laparoscope and other tools. Next, carbon dioxide gas is used to inflate the belly, and this allows me to see the inside of the abdomen in high definition as the surgeon and assistant maneuver the camera around inside. The surgeon then cuts the bile duct and removes the gallbladder. An x-ray called a *cholangiogram* is then used to look for any missed stones. Toward the end of the surgery, I am able to hold the camera rod and even suture the tiny lacerations closed. This is my first suture repair, and my hands are shaking and sweating.

10:30 a.m.

The third surgery is an inguinal hernia repair. During this surgery, I hold the skin back with a retractor and am taught the anatomy up close and personal. My attending surgeon asks me a lot of trivia-like questions, often referred to as *pimping*. This is often part of clinical rotations and is done with good intentions to help students remember information. For example, as he is washing out the wound, he says, "The solution to pollution is . . . ?" expecting me to finish the phrase. The answer is dilution. I missed the first question. The second question is, "What are the layers of the anterior abdominal wall?" The answer is the skin, superficial and deep fascia, the rectus abdominis muscle, external and internal oblique muscles, the transverse abdominal muscle, the fascia transversalis, and the peritoneum. He didn't expect me to know this one, but I'm sure he'll ask me again later.

11:30 a.m.

We took a lunch break in the doctors' lounge, and then Chris and I start rounding on all the postoperative patients in the hospital. I am shocked to hear that one of the postoperative questions I had to ask our patients was, "Are you passing gas yet?" I can't think of a more awkward question. I learn that it is important because if you are unable to pass gas, it could lead to the postoperative complication ileus, otherwise known as intestinal obstruction.

3 p.m.

A patient comes into the emergency department (ED) with a pneumothorax, air or gas in the lining around the lung (pleural cavity). She has not been responding to the chest-tube treatment given in the ED because there is a persistent air leak from the lung. The surgery team is consulted to evaluate for the need for a procedure called a *pleurectomy* to seal the air leak. The surgery begins as a video-assisted thoracoscopic (VATS) pleurectomy, but unfortunately, due to existing adhesions, it is converted to an open *thoracotomy*. My attending surgeon cuts an opening in the cartilage just above the rib and retracts the ribs apart to expose the damaged lung. I catch a glimpse of the heart beating in its pericardial sac. This is all possible because the anesthesiologist has control of the air in and out of the lungs. When the lung is collapsed, it is easier to see the lung and the pleural cavity. After the surgery, the chest is closed, and two chest tubes are placed. The tips of the tubes are placed into a sealed container under water to form an airtight drainage system.

5 p.m.

I experienced four different surgeries today and also rounded on 20 postoperative patients, learning about various postoperative complications. Tonight I need to take notes on the questions I was asked and the correct answers, study the gallbladder anatomy, and look up what ERCP stands for.

In the classroom, I was always amazed at how the body worked. Every detail is so intricate and woven together so perfectly to make a functioning human being. Reading and seeing pictures in books is one thing, but being in the OR and seeing all the parts of the body functioning as a unit is completely different—it's amazing!

A DAY IN THE LIFE: PEDIATRIC PA STUDENT ROTATION

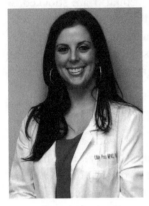

Elizabeth Poss, MPAS, PA-C

6:30 a.m.

Lub-dub, lub-dub; my heart beats with intensity and excitement; as I make my way down an unending abyss of white walls fragrant with the scent of hand sanitizer. Each hallway brings a door with a pin code and finally I reach my destination: the resident's room. I see the flashing in the keypad of the door, assuring me that I am in the correct place.

I am anxious to see what this next month will hold as I enter the world of in-patient pediatrics as a second-year PA student. I meet my chief resident. He introduces me to the residents and medical students and outlines my job responsibilities. I will be writing progress notes on admitted patients, writing history and physical examination (H&P) notes on new patients, and performing.

My first three patients are H&Ps, and thankfully, I finish in the allotted time period. Now it's time to present. Eager with anticipation, I begin my first presentation: a 4-year-old boy with a 5-day history of irritability, fever, *conjunctivitis*, and *desquamation* on his palms. I am immediately cut off by the chief resident and asked to "get to the point" of my assessment and plan. Taken aback, I promptly make my point. I presume that by the end of this rotation I will have the sharpest and timeliest presenting skills in all of Los Angeles.

9:00 a.m.

The attending arrives and everyone stands to attention as though our fearless leader has finally returned to establish order. He is calm and gentle, unlike the intense chief resident. We begin rounds. Our first patient is a 4-day-old boy with a total bilirubin level of 18.5. I am called on and asked to explain the differentials for hyperbilirubinemia. I spout off what I can recall from months ago and pray that I covered enough material. Apparently, these answers have sufficed for now, but I know that I will constantly need to be on my "A" game come 9 a.m. every morning. After reviewing the patients on the floor, we head to the pediatric intensive-care unit (PICU).

9:30 a.m.

The first patient is a 15-year-old girl from Nicaragua who has had three seizures in the last 24 hours. Initially, seizure activity involved only right arm tremors, which progressed to full-blown tonic-clonic seizures. After doing a CT scan, a diagnosis of neurocysticercosis is made. We all clamor around to see the image of the "scolex" (the anterior or headlike portion of a tapeworm) and feel like we are looking straight into a textbook. It is unreal.

The next patient is a 4-year-old boy with a skull fracture. He said while riding his bike when he saw some butterflies and closed his eyes briefly to "fly with them"—and consequently fell into head dive on to the pavement. He was not wearing a helmet. These endearing experiences of innocence remind me why I love children and how special it is to share in their care and their lives.

Shortly after rounding on all the patients, we are brought back to the resident room and begin updating the patient log, getting discharge papers in order, and adding new plans and orders for patients who need further workup. Before the chief resident starts asking me difficult medical questions, he tells me, "You will hate me, but by the end of this, you will thank me." I personally enjoy the challenge of answering these questions; this propels me to keep learning. He is reminding me why I need to know as much as possible and how to become a great clinician, so I take him for his word. Thus I begin researching differential diagnoses for sterile *pyuria* and somogyi effect versus dawn phenomenon.

In the arduous task of doing research, I also become cognizant of my status within the confines of these white walls and take a moment to reflect. As a student, you are always the low person on the totem pole, In being somewhat of the underdog, there is pride in proving yourself and earning the respect of those around you. This rotation, like so many others, is recognition of working hard and making the most of your abilities in this great career.

12:00 Noon

Ah, lunch! The medical student and I quickly whiz through the crowded cafeteria and scan our $8 worth of food and rush back to lunch lecture.

Today's topic is diabetes and other endocrine disorders in the pediatric population. This is probably the thing I love most about this rotation. The learning never ends, and there are a plethora of resources to draw from. The beauty of being a student is the fact that you get to take advantage of every learning opportunity to broaden your knowledge and learn.

3:00 p.m.

The shift has ended for my colleagues and for the medical student, and I am getting ready to tackle the 36-hour call shift with one of the interns. We bravely face the night and get ready for the cases that will catapult our caffeine drive into the wee hours.

5:00 p.m.

The evening begins with a 7-year-old girl with a supracondylar fracture after falling on her outstretched arm in a "Bounce House." She will be admitted to the floor to await surgery later tonight. I pay her a visit, looking for signs of *compartment syndrome*. She has good capillary refill and shows no signs of severe swelling. She is anxious to leave and wants to know when she can go home and play.

7:00 p.m.

We admit a 5-year-old boy for acute appendicitis. His pain is poorly controlled, so we prescribe more pain medication while waiting for the surgery team to see him. I add him to the patient log and anticipate more cases for the evening.

10:00 p.m.

"Every time a bell rings an angel gets his wings." This infamous line from *It's a Wonderful Life* bears some relation to the chimes that we hear in the hospital. I have learned this chime heard over the loud speaker is a baby gracing us with his or her arrival into the world. This sound seems slightly less angelic as we approach the early-morning hours. I go with the intern to the second floor, where mothers and babies are recovering, to do newborn examinations and discharge paperwork. I silently hope to make an indentation on the on call room's pillow soon.

12:00 Midnight

I get my wish and sleep for 2 hours and am awakened to help with the H&P of a 3-month-old girl admitted for an apparent life-threatening event (ALTE). The full workup is ordered, and the patient is placed in the PICU for observation. Now I get to go back to sleep for another quick nap.

6:30 a.m.

I have survived 24 hours and still have 12 more to go. Despite this, I am thankful to have the opportunity to work long shifts because it means less commute time. I am reminded why I love the career choice I've made to become a PA! I appreciate the ability to practice medicine and freedom of choice when it comes to lifestyle, according to my chosen specialty. Pediatrics has given me an appreciation for the beauty of life—a simple smile, the joy of a high five, and the miracle of God working through us to provide healing and answers to very sick children. I will treasure this experience and let it lead me to a lifetime of success.

A DAY IN THE LIFE: REALITY OF STUDENT ROTATIONS

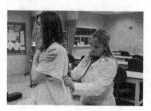

Alexandra Godfrey, BSc, PT, PA-C

In my hand lie the fingers of a dead man, blanched white and icy cold, awaiting dissection. This morning in gross anatomy lab we are studying the tissues of the forearm and hand. I have body 1, a man who died 6 months ago. I don't know the cause of his death, but as I examine his body, I see lungs coated black, a heart stitched with blue, and fingers clubbed and yellow. I formulate a diagnosis, imagining diaphoresis, Levine's sign, and tombstones. I cut the skin shoulder to hand, revealing a delicate cobweb of tissue and a swath of musculature. I examine the muscle layers of his posterior forearm. I marvel at the multitude of tendons running wrist to hand. When I pull on his abductor pollucis, he gives me the thumbs up, and I wonder if he is happy with my work. I hope so. I have found gross anatomy difficult: I held this man's brain, tried to see the soul in the mush, and placed the gray matter in a Ziploc bag. I determined not to forget that moment. He left a legacy that I intend to honor—my brain studying his brain, his right hand in mine, guiding my future practice as a PA.

Morning

Later that morning, I see tombstones on an electrocardiogram (ECG). In clinical medicine, we are studying cardiology. The instructor is a cardio-thoracic PA from a local hospital. He is passionate about his subject: first-degree, second-degree, third-degree block. Wenckebach and Mobitz are my soul mates, helping me decipher the heart's cryptic code. As a class, we are learning to trace life. The PA teaches us segment by segment, wave by wave, building our knowledge and future potential: ventricular depolarization is QRS, *repolarization* is T, and ST-segment elevation with downward concavity creates a frown. I think about body 1: What was his expression? The class continues, and the PA starts to quiz us, searching for proof of our knowledge rather than the heart's reflection. The room pulses with energy as we call out the answers to the instructor's questions. No one wants to be pimped—not now, not ever at the end. We learn about dys-rhythmias: couplets, salvo, and torsades de pointes. I think of ballet as the points of my ECG calipers skip from P to R and jump the QRS. The dance stops at asystole; we check the leads, the connections, the monitor, the power, and the patient's pulse. Cardiopulmonary resuscitation (CPR) begins; we call the code, but it is noon and time has run out.

Early Afternoon

At 1:10 p.m. I watch my preceptor pronounce death. I am on a site visit at a nearby hospital. My plan was to perform a history and physical examina-tion on a patient in the ICU. I was ready to practice my newly acquired skills, but instead, I am examining death again. I met my preceptor (an ICU PA) 10 minutes ago; she flew through the doors of the ICU, instruct-ing me to follow her because she had a death to pronounce downstairs and a patient coding upstairs. I ran down the stairs with her, listening as she explained the status of her two patients. When we arrived on the lower floor, she slowed her pace, signaling to me to wait by the entrance of her patient's room.

The room is bright, lit by the midday sun. A man lies propped on pil-lows in the bed. The etchings of time mark his face; vaults and niches have replaced muscle and fat. Three women stand guard over the patient, anxiously watching and waiting. My preceptor pulls out her stethoscope to auscultate the patient's chest, moving as if she has an infinite amount of time, searching aortic to mitral, listening for tones in a silent heart. I look away for a moment, thinking that this asystole is death run amok; naivety and classroom squashed in favor of a direct line to the ultimate solution. No medicine for this. No hope of curing. The monitor is off, CPR was never started, and I am powerless. I had not considered this possibility when I studied the physical examination of the cardiac and pulmonary systems. Did I miss this section of the checklist?

When I look back, my preceptor nods to the women, confirming that this is indeed the end of life. They crumple. She speaks to them of beginnings and endings—birth, life, and death. The sun shines on. The women cry silently, listening to my preceptor and visibly soothed by the meaning she instills in the moment. One by one, the women approach, thanking her for her work and rewarding her kindness with their hugs, tears, and words of admiration. I watch as a woman strokes the hair and then caresses the face of the body, as women do and will do to infinity. She whispers in his ear, speaking of love, life, and times immemorial. My preceptor moves slowly out of the room, stopping to tuck the blankets up under her patient's chin. I follow her out of the unit. She breaks into a run. We ascend the stairs two at a time. At the top, the phone rings in her pocket. It is the neurosurgeon: No more CPR for the patient upstairs; his brain has collapsed, leaving no structure to examine or lines to trace. This end is precocious, transcending the boundaries set by both medicine and culture. At 30 years old, this man has defied expectations and disintegrated beyond the form of even body 1.

Young death looks quite different. No etchings on this face, just a scattering of pale brown macules across the nose. I see the bulk of the biceps, triceps, and temporalis and then think about the atrophy of bodies 1 and 2. This face is ashen, but the chest moves, and the fingers are warm. With eyes half shut, this young man looks as if he is caught between waking and sleeping. The monitor, the power, and the ventilator are still on. A flat line runs across the screen. Shock and surprise govern the experience.

Moments ago my preceptor had told the family that their son, brother, father had reached the end of his life. She told the mother first, bringing her forward in her wheelchair away from the family group in the waiting area. As she spoke of hypoxia, irreversible brain damage, and asystole, the rest of the family tiptoed forward to listen. They whirled back, their brains in turmoil as they rejected the diagnosis, only to advance again as if wanting, yet not wanting, to know the truth—a *danse macabre*. My preceptor gathered the family together, ushering them to the patient's room and motioning to me to wait by the door.

Again, I watch death from the wings. The choreography differs slightly: A nurse exits the room, sinks against the wall, and sighs, "I feel so bad for this family." The patient's sister looks over at me and whispers, "I cannot believe this is happening." I nod to both. The family fills the room, all standing at least 6 feet from the bed. Eventually, the mother rises from her wheelchair, steps forward, and reaches for her son. Her movements are tremulous, muscles quivering, hands shaking, yet her spirit holds. My preceptor rushes to support her, placing her hand on the mother's arm, guiding her safely toward her son. The rest of the family follows her, forming a body of unity around the man in the bed. My preceptor leaves quietly, stopping to inform me that now it is time for me to meet my patient. It is 3 p.m., and I feel exhausted.

Late Afternoon

My patient looks tired, too. He gives me a weary smile as I walk into the room. My preceptor introduces us, and I start my history and physical examination. I carefully establish my patient's chief complaint and history of presenting illness. Once I have listened to his story, I pull out my stethoscope, listening aortic to mitral, hearing murmurs of the days to come. I think about my patient's 80 pack-year smoking history, wondering if his lungs are already coated black. Fine crackles and expiratory wheezes confirm my suspicion that this man's tissues are already succumbing to disease. I know his story: A virus is destroying his immune system, creating havoc where there was once order and synchrony. His CD4 count is 111, his lungs are awash with *PCP*, and his heart is failing.

When my patient tires, I settle at the desk in his room and examine his charts. The sun is setting, and the day is coming to an end. The room is dimly lit, but I work by the light emanating from the hallway. After a short while, my patient stirs from his sleep and calls me to his bedside. As I stand by him, he reaches his hand out and says, "Alexandra, I am not ready to die." I pause, stopping to think about the hand of body 1, the face of body 2, and the sudden death of body 3—each human a mystery but each teaching me a little more about medicine and its practice. I look at my patient's monitor and see the QRS hop-skip across the screen. I think about my preceptor—words spoken, hands touched, sheets tidied. I take my patient's outstretched hand, wrap his fingers in mine, and say, "I know."

Acknowledgment: This piece of writing is dedicated to the memory of Lara Rutan, a PA whose kindness, compassion, and generosity brightened the lives of so many.

At the time of this writing, **Alexandra Godfrey** was a second-year student in the PA program at Wayne State University, Detroit, MI.

Reprinted, with permission, from the *Journal of the American Academy of Physician Assistants*, October 2009.

[CHAPTER 5]

Transition from School to Work

FINANCIAL PREPARATION

The time period between completing your training and your first paycheck may take up to six months. In that time, you need to study and pass the National Board Examination, apply for a National Provider Identifier (NPI) number and a Drug Enforcement Administration (DEA) number, research jobs, and attend interviews. The board examination costs $475, the DEA license costs $731, and state licensure costs $200 to $300. The NPI number is free.

Once you have found a job and signed a contract, you may need to apply for hospital privileges. In a hospital-based job, you cannot work until you receive approval from the hospital committee, and this process alone can take up to six months. Knowing this information ahead of time will help you to budget money while in physician assistant (PA) school. Ideally, you should have six months of living costs set aside by the time you finish school.

Financial Planning

In your first year of practice, it is wise to live like a starving student. Experience what it feels like to work hard and save. When you see your first paycheck, you may be surprised at how much money comes out in the form of taxes. If your written contract states that you earn $100,000, you will likely take home around $60,000. If you are a Form 1099 independent contractor, you pay taxes four times a year. Form W2 employers will contribute toward taxes with each paycheck. State and federal laws vary. The Internal Revenue Service (IRS) has guidelines that you and your tax adviser should examine.

Consider investing in a Roth individual retirement plan (IRA) prior to the start of your new job because the ability to contribute is based on your annual income. The maximum contribution is $5,000 per year, but as your salary increases, the money you are allowed to contribute decreases. If you or your household (combined spousal income) makes over $183,000 annually, you are unable to contribute or start a Roth IRA. A household that makes more than $183,000 still can invest in a retirement fund (e.g., a 401k) but not a Roth IRA. Roth contributions are not tax deductible, and qualified distributions are tax-free—unlike a traditional 401k retirement account.

Here is an example of a way for a household to be eligible to invest in both types of retirement funds (401k and Roth IRA) if the combined household income is $200,000. If both husband and wife each make $100,000 and each give the maximum amount into his or her 401k, which is $17,000 per year, or $34,000 total, that would decrease their combined income to $166,000 ($200,000 − $34,000 = $166,000). This would now make them eligible to invest in a Roth IRA because their combined income is now considered $166,000, which is below the $183,000 cutoff. Another simple option that some companies offer is a Roth 401k, which has no income restrictions. Take the time to explore all retirement-plan options.[1]

Jeff Rose, a certified financial planner, explains the benefits of starting a retirement account at a young age with this scenario. See Table 5-1 comparing two young adults, Super Saver Parker and Super Slacker Sloane.[1] Both are college graduates with high-paying jobs and have enough income to start contributing to a Roth IRA. Super Saver Parker starts putting $2,000 a year into his Roth IRA ($166.67 per month) at age 25. He does this for a total of 10 years and stops when he has put in a grand total of $20,000. Why does he stop? Don't ask. That's just part of the illustration. Super Slacker Sloane puts off saving into his Roth IRA because he wants to "buy stuff." He finally gets it and starts putting $2,000 a year starting at age 35. Wanting to catch Parker, he puts in $2,000 a year for 30 years, contributing $60,000 in total—$40,000 more than Parker. *We're assuming that they both average 8 percent return on their money.* Who will have more money at age 65?

The person who started 10 years earlier actually made *$73,633 more, even though investing $40,000 less.* The moral of the story is save early and save often. The beauty of the Roth IRA is that your earnings in the end are tax-free.[1]

Table 5-1. Comparison of Savings Plans of Super Saver Parker and Super Slacker Sloane

Super Saver Parker	10 Years of Contributions	Super Slacker Sloane	30 Years of Contributions
25	$2,000	25	—
26	$2,000	26	—
27	$2,000	27	—
28	$2,000	28	—
29	$2,000	29	—
30	$2,000	30	—
31	$2,000	31	—
32	$2,000	32	—
33	$2,000	33	—
34	$2,000	34	—
35	—	35	$2,000
36	—	36	$2,000
37	—	37	$2,000
38	—	38	$2,000
39	—	39	$2,000
40–65	—	40–65	$50,000
Total contributions	$20,000		$60,000
Ending account value	$340,060		$266,427
BIG difference		$73,633	

Source: Reproduced, with permission, from J. Rose, "The Roth IRA Movement: Over 140 Bloggers Doing Their Part to Promote Savings." Good Financial Cents, March 27, 2012; available at: www.goodfinancialcents.com/roth-ira-account-movement/.

Job Search

Prior to the job search, make yourself marketable. Update your curriculum vitae (CV), and have a PA review it to give you feedback. Research the job market in your geographic location. Know the state laws and reimbursement and salary ranges. Then, identify your goals. Are your immediate, short-term goals to learn, to obtain specialty training, to help people, or to make the most amount of money? What are the long-term goals in your career?[2]

To simplify the job-search decision, there are three key components to consider—people, place, and pay:

1. *People.* Most important, chose a supervising physician who will teach you. Next, consider your working relationship with his or her physician partners, the nursing staff, the office manager, and the patient population.
2. *Place.* Ideally, choose a place that has worked with PAs before. PA-familiar institutions tend to use, pay, and treat PAs better than institutions unfamiliar with PAs. Consider working at a teaching hospital, otherwise known as a university or community hospital. The system and the staff are accustomed to physician residents, who are in your same situation as you, fresh out of school and ready to learn.
3. *Pay.* The geographic location will affect your pay. Some areas pay higher, but don't forget to factor in the local cost-of-living expenses such as housing, utilities, and transportation. Also consider the dollar value of any employer-paid benefits.

There are many different avenues through which to find a job. Examples include online organization job postings, hospital web pages, temporary or full-time employment agencies, conferences, and the old-fashion method of handing in a résumé and asking if there are any available openings.

Conferences are a great resource for networking and getting plugged into the job market. At most conferences, there is an exhibition where vendors or companies display their products or information. Companies that employee PAs will get your information and inform you about upcoming openings at their job sites.

Be sure to use *The PA Job Link*, the American Academy of Physician Assistants (AAPA) official online career center at www.healthecareers .com/aapa//. Links to various articles are posted daily relating to job-search tips, CV and interview etiquette, and social media guidelines. The web page allows you to post your CV and customize your job search. New career opportunities are up to date. A section is dedicated to companies or employers who hire PAs and includes the company's mission statement, contact information, available opportunities, benefits, and location facts. This site also helps you to connect with potential employers at upcoming healthcare events or conferences.

INTERVIEW

Know what you'd like to achieve from this potential job opportunity prior to the interview. Decide your bottom line in the following areas: salary, type of work, hours, and lifestyle. To assist with potential salary negotiations, research the local PA, physician, and nursing salaries prior to the interview. When asked what salary you prefer, you can say, "Based on the research I've done, I believe that my salary range should fall somewhere between _____ and _____." Before you interview, you should know who has the authority to make the final decision for hiring.[2] Interviewing with the physician is critical. If he or she is too busy to interview you and has the office manager do so instead, this can be a red flag.[3]

Bring a copy of your CV, PA program-completion certificate, National Commission on Certification of Physician Assistants (NCCPA) certificate, and a list of references with you to your interview.

Etiquette is the staple behind a good interview. Walk in with confidence, and extend your hand to give a firm handshake while maintaining eye contact. Sit when instructed to do so, and maintain proper posture with shoulders back and leaning slightly forward. Interview coach Carol Martin recommends observing the interviewer's style and pace and then attempting to match that style.[4] Answer each question asked, and if possible, provide an example or story to make your point stand out.

At the end of the interview, when asked if you have any questions, ask questions. This highlights your genuine interest. Executive career coach Meg Montford wrote an excellent article entitled, "Three Good Questions to Ask at a Job Interview."[5] Here they are:

1. Why is this position open? Is it a new position, or did someone leave? If someone left, what was his or her reason? Is there an internal candidate also interviewing?

2. What is the most important (or biggest) problem you have that you want someone in this position to tackle? This question tells the company that you're already processing how you may contribute value to them.

3. How will my performance be evaluated in this position, and by whom? This question tells the company that you are thinking about how you'll be doing your new job and that you are ambitious.

After each interview, be sure to mail a thank-you note to further establish your interest in the position.

WHAT CHARACTERISTICS TO LOOK FOR IN YOUR SUPERVISING PHYSICIAN/ FUTURE EMPLOYER

The interview may be your only opportunity to meet your future supervising physician (SP) before you sign the job contract. This is not enough time to observe this person's characteristics and qualities. Once you have passed the interview, and before you sign the contract, consider spending a workday shadowing your SP to see if this job is the right fit for you. Being around the office also will give you a chance to speak with the office staff, and you can observe the interaction between the SP and his or her staff.

You should have a clear vision of what you are looking for in a physician partner. Make a list of those desired qualities.[3] Honesty, integrity, and respect are characteristics that should be at the top of your list. Ultimately, you want your SP to be the kind of provider you want to become. Try to find someone who is patient and supportive, who can provide the amount of teaching you will require, and who believes in the team approach to medicine.

Jennifer Anne Hohman, AAPA's director of professional advocacy, recommends researching the physician and the practice extensively before accepting a job offer. "Have they worked with PAs before, and if so, how well did they retain them? High turnover is a worrisome sign. Does the practice employ family members? Spouses serving as office managers can create difficult dynamics for PAs, with physicians being reluctant to go to bat for the PA in terms of salary or other contract or practice issues the practice manager opposes."[3]

THINGS TO INCLUDE IN YOUR FIRST JOB CONTRACT

Your contract and delegation-of-services (DOS) agreement should be signed prior to starting your job. The DOS agreement defines the working relationship and delegation of duties between the SP and PA. It typically includes "the prescribing of controlled substances; the degree and means of supervision; the frequency and mechanism of chart review; procedures addressing situations outside the scope of practice of the physician assistant; and procedures for providing backup for the physician assistant in emergency situations."[6] A *contract* is defined as a "legally binding, deliberate and voluntary agreement that is between two or more competent parties, and is evidenced by (1) an offer, (2) acceptance of the offer, and (3) a valid (legal and valuable) consideration."[7] The AAPA website has excellent resources for this process.[8]

Terms of the Contract

The term of your agreement should be clearly stated, including a start and end date and options for contract renewal. Schedule evaluations every six months. In this way, there is potential growth for your PA scope of practice and salary.

There are two types of termination provisions: with cause and without cause. Termination of a contract *with cause* is due to specified serious reasons, for example, violation of part of the agreement, suspension of license, and illicit or illegal behavior. By definition, termination of contract *without cause* is when either party can end the contract at any time without reason. A 90-day notice is usually required.[8]

Compensation

Cleary define the details of compensation. The following questions from AAPA's "Anatomy of a Contract" will help you.

Will you be paid a salary, an hourly rate, a percentage of fees billed or collected or salary plus bonus based on productivity? If your compensation will be based on a percentage of fees billed, specify which fees will be included in the calculation. If you will be paid an hourly rate, include a minimum number of hours per week or per month to ensure adequate income. Terms should be clearly defined in the contract—not only the amount (and/or percentage of productivity income) but also the frequency of calculation and payment. For comparison purposes, find out what colleagues in your area earn from a customized salary profile provided by the AAPA for a nominal fee.[8]

Malpractice Insurance and Disputes

Malpractice insurance can be joint with your SP or separate as your own policy. There are two types of policies: claims-made and occurrence. A *claims-made* policy protects you for claims that *occur and are reported* during the policy period. It is important, then, to purchase *tail coverage*, which will protect you against claims filed after the policy ends. An *occurrence* policy covers you during the policy period regardless of when the claim is made.[8]

In the case of a dispute between you and your employer, be sure that the contract states that you will have access to medical records if a lawsuit is filed against you after you leave the practice. If this clause is lacking in your contract, your lawyer will have to subpoena the records, which costs money and time.[8]

Benefits

Remember that the federal government does not tax benefits. If you have the opportunity to negotiate a higher salary *or* a better benefits package, choose the benefits package. Fringe benefits are benefits received in addition to regular pay. Most PAs receive health insurance, dental insurance, life insurance; retirement plans, paid vacation time, paid continuing medical education (CME) hours, and paid hospital medical staff fees. These benefits should be clearly spelled out in your contract. Other less common benefits can include vision insurance, paid professional dues, licensure fees, books and professional journals, NCCPA fees, and U.S. Drug Enforcement Administration registration fees.[8]

As you wait for your contract to be written up, consider making an appointment with a contract lawyer. It may cost $1,000 up front but can save you thousands of dollars in mistakes down the road. When your contract is handed to you, ask for a week to sign and return it. Research the benefits package extensively, and call the insurance companies. Be sure to read over your contract with an experienced PA who also works in your state. If there are areas of concern, address them.

Jennifer Anne Hohman warns: "Review the contract carefully for highly restrictive noncompete clauses and overly long termination notice periods. If you find yourself in a position that is burning you out, failing to foster your growth, treating you unfairly or engaging in unethical practices, you'll want to move on with grace and professionalism."[3]

Areas of Caution

1. Look into your state laws. For example, Rebecca Issacman, PA-C, warns, "Colorado is an at-will state. You can be hired and fired at the will of the employer without reason or notice."

2. If you sign a contract as an independent contractor, understand what this really means. You will likely have to purchase your own malpractice insurance and take your own taxes out of you pay. Discuss this with your accountant, and a contact lawyer prior to signing this type of contract.

3. A PA who held seven part-time jobs in her first years shares her story: "My first mistake was not making sure a contract was in place before starting work. I actually made this mistake several times. Part-time work became very attractive when I did not have a job. One family-practice doctor I worked for did not show up to see her patients one day. As a brand-new PA with very little experience, I was alone in her office seeing all her patients as well as mine that were scheduled for that day. The following week this scenario played out again. I quit this job after working for one month and was never paid. This was, however, my mistake because a proper contract was not in place."

WHAT PHYSICIANS EXPECT FROM THEIR PHYSICIAN ASSISTANTS AND HOW TO MEET THOSE EXPECTATIONS

It's important to understand the expectations of your SP. It is equally important for you to understand your role in the partnership, as well as the limitations within your scope of practice. Although there are universally accepted expectations regardless of where you work, you'll need to know the different skill sets needed to work in a hospital environment versus a private practice.

All physicians invest time training, developing, and partnering with their PAs. Private-practice physicians also invest a portion of their salary in this partnership. In return, they hope that their PA becomes an extension of them, enabling their practice to see more patients in a given period of time. To become this partner, the PA must be teachable, knowledgeable, and a team player. He or she must be dependable, honest, and hardworking. Patients and physicians alike want a PA who is compassionate, friendly, and a skilled communicator. As with any other occupation, the employer expects the employee to be at his or her "best." "The quality of expectations determines the quality of our action."[9]

Scope of Practice

Always be conscious of your scope of practice, and err on the side of caution. Your SP needs you to be responsible for staying within the DOS boundaries. If you are presented with a patient whose condition exceeds your level of training or experience, ask for help. You are not expected to know everything, but you must know when to ask for help. Communicate this to your SP in a clear and concise way. Say, "I need you to come see this patient because I am unsure," instead of just presenting a patient as you normally would. Communication is vital.

Differences between Private Practice and the Hospital Setting

There are significant differences in physicians' expectations with regard to working in a hospital setting versus a private practice. While working in a hospital setting, you may have a large number of SPs. You must learn the individual doctors' style of treating patients. Your SP is expecting you to be his or her extension and expects excellent communication skills because you are often managing several patients together at the same time.

Being in a hospital setting, you must be able to handle chaotic situations. You are not in a controlled environment with a tidy schedule, seeing one patient at a time. Interruptions are inevitable. For example, you may be seeing a patient and at the same time you get a phone call from your SP, a page from a nurse with a question about another patient, and an in-person request from a consultant physician. Expectations are that you stay organized and calm and that you complete all tasks without error.

Dedication and hard work are top qualities that a SP is going to expect in private practice. Often the PA is expected to be in the office the same hours per week as the SP. Sometimes this means staying late at work finishing paperwork or taking work home with you to complete. Before signing a contract in private practice, understand the expected work hours. It is important to determine if writing progress notes will be done during work hours or if you will be expected to stay after hours finishing that day's progress notes. An experienced PA in private practice warns: "My supervising doctor expected me to be as hard working and dedicated to our patients as he was. That was fine, until he took on more than he could handle. At one point in my life, I felt like all I did was work. My hours were 7 a.m. to 6:30 p.m. I would come home, put my kids to bed by 8 p.m., and work on my charts for up to three hours per night." Another PA states: "I was not prepared for the pace of the facility in my first job. I was required to see a new patient every 15 minutes, which included documentation for each encounter as part of my workflow. I ended up with piles of charts to complete at the end of the day. I was not compensated for my two hours of extra time each day because I was a salaried employee." This goes back to the point made earlier: Decide your bottom line in the area of work hours and lifestyle prior to the start of your job, and include it in your contract.

Contrasting the expectations of a PA working in a hospital environment versus a private practice is meant as an exercise to determine which may best fit your personality and/or needs. With effort and a positive attitude, you will form an excellent rapport with your SP and grow to meet his or her expectations.

Checklist

List of what a new PA needs on the first day of the job:

____ Signed contract and DOS agreement

____ State license

____ NCCPA certification

____ Malpractice insurance

____ Medicare enrollment

____ Medicaid provider number

____ DEA number (if prescribing controlled substances)

____ State controlled substance number (required in some states)

____ Hospital privileges (if working in hospital setting)

Once your start working:

____ Keep track of your CME

____ Keep receipts for all professional expenses

____ Keep a procedure log and periodically have your SP sign it

---

References

1. Rose, J. "The Roth IRA Movement: Over 140 Bloggers Doing Their Part to Promote Savings." *Good Financial Cents*, March 27, 2012; available at: www.goodfinancialcents.com/roth-ira-account-movement/.

2. Goodrich, D. "Lecture on Contracts and CVs." Presented at the AAPA Annual Conference, Toronto, Canada, May 28, 2012.

3. "Finding Dr. Right: What PAs Should Look for in a Physician Partner." *PA Professional Magazine*, September 2011; available at: www.aapa.org.

4. Martin, C. "Three Common Deadly Mistakes Made in Job Interviews." 2012; available at: http://interviewcoach.com/blog/how-to-prevent-these-three-common-deadly-mistakes-in-job-interviews/.

5. Montford, M. "Three Good Questions to Ask at a Job Interview." 2012. Available at: www.healthecareers.com/article/3-good-questions-to-ask-at-a-job-interview/169413.

6. Physician Assistant Act. Part I: General Provisions, 58-70a-102. Definitions: 2b. Title 58, Chap. 70a. Utah Code Annotated 1953. As Amended by Session Laws of Utah 2012. Issued May 8, 2012.

7. www.businessdictionary.com/definition/contract.html

8. American Academy of Physician Assistants. "Anatomy of a Contract." Available at: www.aapa.org/your_pa_career/interviewing_and_contracts/resources/item.aspx?id=2581.

9. A. Godin, French author, 1880–1938.

10. American Academy of Physician Assistants. "From Program to Practice: A Guide to the Physician Assistant Profession." AAPA, 2008, pp. 123–124.

[CHAPTER 6]

Interprofessional Collaboration in Healthcare Delivery

By design, physicians and PAs [physician assistants] work together as a team, and all PAs practice medicine with a physician supervision. Supervision does not mean, though, that a supervising physician must always be present with the PA or direct every aspect of PA-provided care. PAs are trained and educated similarly to physicians and therefore share similar diagnostic and therapeutic reasoning. Physician-PA practice can be described as delegated autonomy. Physicians delegate duties to PAs, and within those range of duties, PAs use autonomous decision making for patient care. This team model is an efficient way to provide high-quality medical care. In rural areas, the PA may be the only healthcare provider on-site, collaborating with a physician elsewhere through telecommunication.[1]

As the physician and PA work together, over time, respect, trust, and rapport are built leading to more autonomy for the PA. An expert in the field, Randy D. Danielsen, PhD, PA-C, highlights five necessary characteristics for a successful physician-PA team. They include mutual respect, communication, recognition of each other's strengths and weaknesses, a mutual understanding of the state statutes that govern supervision and PA practice, and a mutual understanding of the PA's scope of practice.[2]

The competency and success of the physician-PA team are crucial factors to optimize all aspects of patient care. This section will give you an inside look from two viewpoints—a PA's personal experience working as a team with her supervising physician and the supervising physician's personal experience working with his PA.

PA'S PERSPECTIVE WORKING WITH A PHYSICIAN IN A PRIVATE PRACTICE

Jessica Rodriguez Ohanesian, MS, PA-C

Case Presentation with My Attending Physician

Me: This is a 40-year-old woman referred by her primary doctor for a 6-month history of a dry, hacking cough, uncontrolled asthma, and progressive dyspnea on exertion (DOE). The patient states, "I used to be an active person, and now it's hard for me to walk from the car into your office. My cough is so severe that it is causing leakage of urine, and I now have to wear Depends." Over the ensuing months, she has had progressive DOE and asthmatic episodes that have responded to prednisone. Last month, an infiltrate was diagnosed on chest x-ray, and antibiotics were prescribed. The patient denies fever, night sweats, or weight loss. She has not taken any new medications, and she works from home without any obvious occupational exposure. Her past medical history is benign other than adult-onset asthma diagnosed 5 years ago. Until recently, she has been controlled on a long-acting bronchodilator and nasal spray. She has no surgical history, is a lifelong nonsmoker, and has no allergies to medications. On review of her recent lab work, her white blood cell count is elevated at 15 with 17 percent peripheral eosinophils.

Dr. B: What do you appreciate on physical exam, and what is your differential?

Me: Vitals are within normal limits, other than tachycardia with a heart rate of 108, and room air oxygen saturation is 96 percent. She speaks in five-word sentences. Her pulmonary exam reveals scattered late expiratory wheezes with inspiratory crackles at bilateral bases. My differential diagnosis is allergic bronchopulmonary aspergillosis (ABPA), chronic eosinophilic pneumonia (CEP), coccidiomycosis, bronchiectasis, chronic obstructive pulmonary disease (COPD), interstitial lung disease (ILD), and lung cancer. Other unlikely differentials include tuberculosis, other infections, occupational or environmental exposure, and medication side effects.

Dr. B: What workup is required to make the diagnosis?

Me: A repeat complete blood cell count (CBC) with differential, serum IgE and IgM for Aspergillus fumigatus, serum IgG and IgM for coccidiomycosis, an α_1-antitrypsin level, an antinuclear antibody test (ANA) and rheumatoid factor (RF) test, an erythrocyte sedimentation rate (ESR), a skin purified protein derivative (PPD) test, full pulmonary function tests, and a high-resolution computed tomographic (CT) scan of the chest. The patient also may need a bronchoscopy if the diagnosis is still indeterminate.

Dr. B: Order the workup, and have the patient return in 2 weeks.

Case to be continued . . .

My first job out of PA school was the first time for me to put my education into practice and the first time that my physician employer had used a PA. He had seen PAs in action during his residency program, liked the idea, and was ready to use a PA in his practice. His private practice needed help, and he understood the benefits that a PA could bring to his practice without the added cost of hiring a new physician. We shared a goal of showing our patients and his physician colleagues how successful a team approach to medicine could be. In one year's time, we met that goal.

Prior to having a PA, my supervising physician did not have enough hours in the day to maintain his busy practice. He had a thriving sleep medicine and pulmonary clinic, was the intensive care unit (ICU) director at the local hospital, and shared responsibilities for being on call several hours per week. He would often arrive late to clinic because of emergencies in the ICU. Once he arrived to clinic, he gave his full and undivided attention to each patient. Given the time constraints, he fell behind on his charting. This had a domino effect, leading to decreased billing and increased disorganization, making his clinic time burdensome. As I interviewed for the position, there were 60 or more incomplete charts on his desk. Many of these charts were new patient consults, each with the potential of $400 in billable profit.

Once hired, I made it a point to arrive to clinic before Dr. B to review and sign returned labs, CT scans, and biopsy results. By the time he arrived to clinic, I had met with each patient, understood the reason for his or her visit, had performed the review of systems, and had completed their physical exams. I presented each patient to Dr. B, and he went into each room to perform his exam, review the chart, and make the final treatment plans. He discussed each patient with me, and I would dictate the notes for that visit. Our method of having two providers see each patient had many benefits. First, I was able to dictate every chart, which kept the office organized and the billing up to date. Second, the patients felt that they were getting more out of their visit by having two providers see them. Third, Dr. B had less stress and was using his time more effectively. Finally, my assessment skills as a PA were growing based on my ability to see the patient first and independently make my own plan and later review it with Dr. B for his final plan.

The office staff also benefited from having a PA. Instead of calling Dr. B with questions, they had me as an additional resource. The piles of charts on Dr. B's desk disappeared. Lab reports and other pertinent faxes were dealt with in a timely manner. The wait time in the clinic decreased from over an hour to less than 15 minutes.

The ICU and hospital work had a similar flow. The mornings were spent together in the unit. I saw each patient and presented the case; Dr. B made amendments, and I dictated the note. I had the time to talk with the nurses and the patient's family about the patient's progress and expected outcome. In the afternoons, I substituted for Dr. B on rounds on the floor patients, affording Dr. B more time to spend with the unit patients for extra consults and procedures. Within months of working as a team, we had a solid system that led to improved patient care, more timely billing and enhanced net profit return, and an overall improvement in the quality of life for Dr. B.

Looking again at the case, in summary, three components are highlighted: asthma, pulmonary infiltrates on chest x-ray, and peripheral eosinophilia. ABPA is the most common diagnosis that comes to mind, but the patient's serology was negative for *Aspergillus*, and the CT scan did not show bronchiectasis. Churg-Strauss syndrome, otherwise known as *chronic eosinophilic pneumonia* (CEP), was the most likely diagnosis after final workup. Repeat lab tests revealed an ongoing leukocytosis with peripheral eosinophils of 20 percent and an elevated ESR of 95. The pulmonary function test showed a moderate restrictive defect with a reduced diffusing capacity. The CT scan showed dense, patchy infiltrates in the mid-upper lung zones. Bronchoscopy revealed a predominance of eosinophils in the bronchoalveolar-lavage fluid. Treatment for CEP was started with prednisone 60 mg daily for 2 weeks, with a slow taper to the lowest amount that would maintain remission. At the 1-month follow-up appointment, the patient remained on prednisone at 30 mg daily, and her symptoms were 80 percent improved. At the 6-month follow-up, while taking Prednisone at 5 mg daily, the infiltrates on the patient's CT scan resolved, and her pulmonary function improved.

PHYSICIAN'S PERSPECTIVE WORKING WITH A PA IN A PRIVATE PRACTICE

Rajan Bhatia, MD

When I hired Jessi to join my practice, it had grown to a volume of several hundred patients with a waiting list. I was looking for someone who would be able to help with the workload and allow me to bring in more new patients. My goal in the beginning was to find someone who would function as a "physician extender"—to be able to see the follow-up patients and assist with the initial history taking for new patients.

To help prepare Jessi for working in a specialty practice, I spent 3 months working extensively with her on building her skills and knowledge level so that, ultimately, she would feel comfortable seeing my patients independently, and I would feel comfortable trusting her judgment. In our initial training period, our interactions were very much like a medical student and a professor. I assigned readings for her weekends off to enhance what she was learning with hands-on interactions with patients. In turn, I allowed her to see the patients and present them to me so that we could discuss what she was seeing. This allowed me to validate what she was learning so that an essential trust level could be built.

After a year of working together, Jessi had surpassed my initial expectations and goals. She had become particularly excellent with taking histories and performing physical exams. As with any skill, taking the history takes practice to achieve competence. The detail with which some patients can relay their historical information can vary wildly. On one hand, laconic patients can range from being absolutely incapable of contributing information to being not particularly forthcoming with details of their histories. On the other hand, there are those "chatterbox" patients who are worried about leaving something out and therefore provide a lot of information that is not relevant to the reason you are seeing them. The art of taking a history is the ability to find a middle ground. To be able to ignore distracting and irrelevant details while being savvy enough to ask the right questions that elicit information that some may not realize is important when forming a diagnosis and plan. Jessi excelled in this and, as a result, also was exceptionally good with the creation of treatment plans that would be most successful for the patient. Her pulmonary diagnostic ability surpassed that of many internists I've known.

The formation of a strong relationship between a PA and physician relies on a few key but *simple* components: adequate training/education/orientation of the PA and clear communication and expectation on both sides. My experience was really positive, and I found that having a PA enriched my practice and allowed me to provide better care to more patients. I would encourage other physicians to look at welcoming a PA into their practice.

PA'S PERSPECTIVE WORKING WITH PHYSICIANS IN EMERGENCY MEDICINE

Jessica Rodriguez Ohanesian, MS, PA-C

Case Presentation with My Attending Physician

Me: This is a 34-year-old man here for hallucinations and insomnia for 3 to 4 days. He has self-doubt and enhanced, racing, accusatory, and persecutory thoughts without suicidal or homicidal idealities. He denies illicit drug or recent steroid use. He has a known history of major depression, without a history of psychosis, and multiple medical problems, including colitis requiring immunosuppressant drugs. Owing to a recent prolonged hospitalization, he also has deep-vein thrombosis (DVT). Vital signs are within normal limits. The patient appears distracted but otherwise is cooperative and answers questions appropriately. His physical exam is within normal limits. My plan is to get a complete blood count, chemistry panel, liver function tests, and a urine toxicology screen.

Attending: Is he still on Coumadin for the DVT?

Me: Yes, he is still on Coumadin. The DVT was diagnosed 5 months ago. I'll add a PT/INR to the blood work.

Attending: What is your differential diagnosis?

Me: My differential diagnosis is depression with psychotic features versus bipolar with depressive features, medication reaction, illicit drug overdose, electrolyte abnormality, uremia/liver failure, with a low suspicion for meningitis/encephalitis. He is anticoagulated, so I think he would be too high risk for a lumbar puncture right now.

Attending: When the medical workup is complete, consult the social worker, and we can touch base again.

Case to be continued . . .

Physician assistants have a 30-year employment history in the teaching hospital where I currently work and accepted my second job as a PA. Many specialties throughout the hospital use PAs, who work alongside medical residents providing a similar level of care. I transitioned from a small private hospital with one supervising physician (SP) to a large teaching hospital with over 35 SPs. Working with so many SPs adds a whole new challenge because it involves remembering each SP's practice style and personal vexations. Some prefer formal and complete patient presentations and then closely follow every detail in the course of the patient's workup, whereas others prefer less formal one-line summary patient presentations including the plan of care for the patient and allow an experienced PA to be more independent.

The hospital's emergency department (ED) is the size of a football field and is one of the largest EDs in the state of California. The ED is staffed with over 300 nurses, 40 medical residents, 35 attending physicians, and 10 PAs. It is divided into six different zones and holds 120 beds. Patients are triaged into the zones by their triage score or level of acuity. PAs work in two of the six zones and work side by side with the medical residents. The attending physicians staff these zones and supervise residents and PAs simultaneously.

The ED is required to care for every person who walks through the doors regardless of their chief complaint or their ability to pay. Free access to medical care, the quality of attention given by the ED staff, and shelter from the outdoor conditions keep the waiting room very busy. There are often 50 or more patients waiting to be seen at one time, with wait times ranging from 2 to 15 hours. Sick patients are often sitting among the "frequent-flyer system abusers," and tempers often flare as patients become angry and frustrated.

During an average day, the PA provider prioritizes the order in which he or she sees patients based on acuity and wait time. The PA reviews the patient's existing medical record, greets the patient, takes a full medical history, and performs the physical exam. The PA then organizes the information, develops a differential diagnosis (a list of possible diagnoses), and a plan for workup and treatment of the patient. The attending physician listens to the PA's presentation of the case and performs an abbreviated physical exam, and together they make a final plan of the necessary workup and treatment. Once the initial medical workup is complete, the PA and SP go back to the drawing board, reevaluating the differential diagnosis and deciding on the most likely diagnosis and best treatment plan. The most important factor from an ED perspective is to rule out life-threatening conditions.

Social workers in the ED assist the medical providers by taking time to talk to patients and their families, which improves patients' quality of life and avoids unnecessary social admissions. Looking back at the case, the social worker believed that the patient needed to have his medications readjusted and that the hallucinations and insomnia could have been induced by the newly prescribed medication. Since this occurred over the weekend, the social worker made a note to call the patient's psychiatrist on Monday.

Looking over the differential diagnosis helped to identify that the symptoms were likely due to depression with psychotic features, bipolar disorder with depressive features, or a medication reaction. The patient also could have new-onset schizophrenia. The labs ruled out life-threatening medical causes, including electrolyte abnormality, drug overdose, and kidney or liver failure. Throughout the patient's ED stay, there was ongoing low suspicion for meningitis or encephalitis. For the patient's comfort, I prescribed a benzodiazepine medication to take before bedtime until he could see his psychiatrist.

PHYSICIAN'S PERSPECTIVE WORKING WITH A PA IN EMERGENCY MEDICINE

Michael D. Burg, MD, FACEP

Colleagues—an emergency physician and a PA—both care for a patient in the emergency department (ED). At intake, the physician does a brief history and physical exam, orders a basic workup, and begins therapy. The PA sees the patient in a treatment area, completes the history and physical exam, compiles the workup results, augments the diagnostic evaluation as necessary, assesses the patient's response to therapy, and arranges an appropriate disposition. The PA and the physician confer as needed during their patient's ED course.

A patient needing a urologic consultation is seen by a PA, who, in turn, discusses the case with her supervising physician. Together, they decide on the proper course of action for their patient.

An orthopedic patient presenting with a difficult hip dislocation is seen simultaneously by a PA and a physician. While the physician manages the patient's pain and prepares for procedural sedation, the PA prepares for a hip reduction. Later, the physician directs medication administration, which facilitates sedation, while the PA performs the procedure.

These vignettes—all taken from real-world experience—represent variations on the theme of teamwork, the norm in most of medicine and a trend that is here to stay.

Physician-PA teamwork fits well with the general concept that medicine can be thought of as a team sport. Teams of hospitalists all care for the same patients. A trauma team mobilizes and responds when a critically injured motor vehicle crash victim is brought to the ED. Multidisciplinary teams—PAs, administrators, pharmacists, nurses, physicians, and others— all round together. And so it is for physician-PA teams. They work together to provide excellent medical care, better than either could supply single-handedly.

It's good for all concerned. The burden of having to know it all and do it all is lifted. Patients benefit from the dual expertise and shared responsibilities brought by their physician-PA team. Specialized knowledge and skill are combined synergistically. Knowledge sharing and learning are enhanced by a team approach to patient care. It's easy to imagine that patient outcome and satisfaction are enhanced as well. After all, as is often said, two heads are better than one. And finally, who really wants to work alone? Being the member of a smoothly functioning, effective healthcare team makes the workday more rewarding and enjoyable. Who wouldn't want that?

Medicine is, and will continue to be, a team sport. PA-MD stands for physician assistant–medical doctor. Going forward, it also may be short for "practice alongside many doctors" (and they alongside you as you move through your career).

PHYSICIAN–PA RELATIONSHIP

Susanne Spano, MD

What is the PA's role in the delivery of health care? This is the question I had when transitioning from medical school into a residency in emergency medicine. My medical school training exemplified an old-fashioned view of medical education, with wizened white-coated men leading a covey of trainees in and out of patient rooms, none of whom were PAs. In that setting, there were scores of medical students, over 200 per class, as well as residents, fellows, and allied health professionals all training together in an unspoken institutional hierarchy where everyone knew what was expected of them and what their contribution to the team was expected to be. The addition of a new piece to the puzzle, the PA, was an enigma to me.

Rotations through medical and surgical specialties presented seemingly inconsistent relationships with PAs in the clinical setting. A theoretical trauma patient presenting to the ED in septic shock would be stabilized and referred to a surgical service, where a surgery PA would likely insert a central venous catheter, perform an arterial puncture for lab tests, and start medications to support the blood pressure. If the patient decompensates despite those methods and definitive surgical care is deemed necessary, the patient is taken to the operating room, intubated by a nurse anesthetist, and sent to recover in the ICU, where a trauma PA floats a Swan-Ganz pulmonary artery catheter. The underlying trauma requires reduction and splinting of bone fragments by an orthopedic PA.

Consideration of the scope of practice for the attending physician providers in each specialty reframes the anticipated role of a PA in that specialty. In most specialties employing PAs, the high volume of patients awaiting care has outpaced the ability of a limited pool of physicians to address those needs. In each specialty mentioned earlier, PAs are often placed in the role of "physician extenders," addressing issues determined by each specialty. Placing an intracranial bolt monitor is a procedure that is outside the scope of physicians from most specialties yet is a routine procedure for neurosurgery PAs. Neurosurgeons want to free up their limited time to be able to perform neurosurgeries, which no other specialist can do, rather than be tied up in the ED placing relatively routine bolt monitors. However, as with the placement of intracranial bolts by neurosurgery PAs, the need for physician extenders in emergency medicine is crucial owing to the high volume of patients seen through an ED. Emergency medicine physicians are required to abruptly stop low-acuity patient care for the emergent pediatric resuscitation, adult cardiac arrest, or multisystem-trauma victim. These dramatic, procedure-rich resuscitations are a small percentage of the emergency physician's case load yet the predominant focus of their training. Given limited human resources, the advent of the PA drastically improves patient flow and efficiency in many departments of medicine.

The PA's role in delivering consistent, high-quality, and cost-effective care is becoming the face of modern healthcare. An ideal physician-PA relationship is cooperative and collegial and should be one of clear expectations. Expectations for the role of a PA in the physician-PA team can be based on the "bread-and-butter model" of each medical specialty, so a procedurally rich career as a PA is best found in the surgical subspecialties, whereas the longitudinal patient-care relationship is best evidenced in primary-care careers. The continuum of medical education is such that physicians train PAs, and in many cases PAs train resident physicians. The decision to embrace a PA career with these specifics in mind is one that can be rewarding and provide lifelong intellectual satisfaction.

SAY ANYTHING: PHYSICIAN-PA RELATIONSHIP

Rais Vohra, MD

When I look back to all the wonderful and rewarding interactions I have had among my professional relationships, I can honestly say that many of them have been with PA providers. Although I have moved cities and jobs several times in the course of my residency, fellowship, and subsequent employment, I continue to value and learn from PAs, whom I work with on an almost daily basis, and I am glad to say that I have stayed friends with those with whom I no longer work. Thus it is a wonderful (and somewhat daunting) opportunity for me to be asked to describe for future PAs the qualities and traits that are most valuable in the physician-PA relationship. I suppose one place to begin is to briefly describe a few PAs I have known.

One PA I've known for a number of years is best deemed a social anthropologist. She is constantly doing "field work," braving uncharted territories of diverse cultures, unusual belief systems, and fragmented or disrupted thought processes of the people we meet and treat in our busy emergency department (ED). And like a real anthropologist coming home from exotic continents and faraway nations, she comes back from her forays into the lives and backgrounds of her patients wiser and worldlier—full of clinical insights and personal narratives that the rest of us could never have gleaned in the daily grind of our own relatively more impoverished attempts at the history and physical exam. For this reason, even though I have more years of experience in the department, I remain a pupil when I watch her work out the real causes and complications of someone's chief complaint. This type of deep, sometimes unconventional, investigation has proved rewarding because it allows us as providers to examine and understand the world of a patient beyond the sterile corridors of the hospital and follow our patient's journey into the streets and homes where much—if not most—of the real work of healing actually takes place.

Yet another PA in our group is a detective. A real gumshoe, he has been doing emergency care through several decades of dramatic changes in our field, and like many veteran detectives on television cop shows, he is constantly and most happily at work when identifying and solving mysteries. His indomitable spirit of inquiry; his courage to ask uncomfortable, tedious, or trivial questions that reveal some key tidbit of vital information from the patients, paramedics, or relatives; and his high standards for himself and others to "do the right thing" for the care of an ill or unfortunate patient are truly inspiring to me. I am glad to be in the company of this real-life modern-day Sherlock of the ED. Through him, I have come to appreciate that the most central quality in "quality improvement" is to never stop learning, whether it is book knowledge or street knowledge, about how patients live, think, and survive through adversities great and small.

A third PA is someone I first met on her first shift out of PA school. Bright-eyed and eager to learn the tips, tricks, and pearls of clinical medicine from those much senior to her in experience, she brought to that first shift an infectious enthusiasm and contagious smile, and this wonderful energy has continued to aid and nurture the development of her clinical knowledge and skill set. Although I never quite heard her say it outright, I surmise that she figured out early in training the secret to success in clinical medicine—optimism blended with compassion.

I recall all these wonderful providers—and I could easily name many others—because of all the great times we had together even while on busy, chaotic, and sometimes stressful shifts in emergency medicine. We taught each other, and we learned together about patients and their diseases, people and their frailties as well as their untapped resilience. As you can see from these very brief vignettes, they are all different people and have very different styles of working. This variety makes my job as an attending physician an exciting one because I am constantly interacting with providers who bring different worldviews, talents, and skill sets to the department. (And I am sure they feel the same about the many different styles of practice that physicians themselves purvey.) What ties all our diverse and equally gifted personalities together? What is the secret to the success of a physician-PA relationship? What, if anything, can serve as a watchword and foundation of the vital bond between all sorts of different providers in the front lines of medical care? What's the glue that unites all these complex and independent elements in the chaos and buzz of clinical medicine?

If I had to choose a single key word, it would definitely have to be *communication*. One of the enduring skills of successful medical practitioners—whether it is a physician, a PA, or anyone who interacts with patients daily—is their well-honed capacity to listen and respond to a variety of patients and relatives, nursing and ancillary staff, and physicians within and beyond the ED. This takes practice and patience, and because communication is the way we all ultimately find out about our patients, their diseases, and their best treatments, it remains the foundation to the constant process of learning and relearning that medicine requires. Beyond the daily practical issues, communication lets us know that there are others who think about the same important and profound questions about life and career and allows us to become valuable and productive members of our communities.

What Freud called the "talking cure" and countless social scientists, medical scholars, and clinical workplace monitors call "effective networking" can even more easily be summarized by two simple words, "Say anything." I think that being able to speak freely to, with, and about the people you work with and around is an underestimated and underemphasized characteristic for a successful workplace relationship regardless of the details of where and how one practices. And because physicians and PAs work so much in sync with each other, this vital and open exchange of ideas, information, insights, and experience is one of the most important relationships that can occur in both their medical careers. Open communication lays the groundwork for genuine respect and mutual trust. And it builds friendships and professional bonds that last the tests of time, distance, and unpredictable factors that inevitably pop up in every department of every hospital.

So, my advice to those who are developing a style and structure to their clinical practice is to go ahead, "Say anything." Be compassionate and polite but also honest to yourself and others around you, especially in the formative months and years when you are still looking for a more permanent place within the diverse and many-chambered house of modern medicine. There is no one way to do emergency medicine or any other specialty, for that matter, as far as I can gather. What is important is that you find a place to practice that allows you to be truly your best self. And when you find an environment where you feel you can be your genuine, true self, you will have arrived at a place worth calling your home base. This is what PAs have taught me with their uplifting, optimistic, and constantly humane approaches to care and why I look forward to my shifts working alongside them in our department.

References

1. "What Is a PA?" American Academy of Physician Assistants website, www.aapa .org/the_pa_profession/what_is_a_pa.aspx (accessed February 1, 2013).

2. Danielsen, R. D. "What Factors Are Necessary for a Successful PA/MD Relationship?" *Medscape Family Medicine*, March 11, 2002; available at: www .medscape.com/viewarticle/429407.

[CHAPTER 7]

Endless Opportunities

A DAY IN THE LIFE: PULMONARY, SLEEP, AND CRITICAL-CARE PA RESIDENCY

Jessica Rodriguez Ohanesian, MS, PA-C

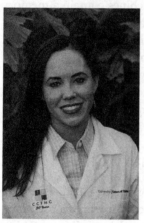

At age 23, I graduated from the Western University Physician Assistant (PA) Program. While job shopping, I came across a pulmonary, sleep, and critical-care private practice with three physicians who were looking for a "green PA" to train for their practice. This practice and the affiliated hospital were about to work with a PA for the first time.

These physicians had completed undergraduate school, medical school, residency, and fellowship totaling 14 years of schooling after high school. I had completed 6 years of schooling. They decided that they would create a "1-year residency" for me. My first 3 months I shadowed, took notes, read, and did minipresentations on related medical topics. During that time, I wrote letters and went to meetings with hospital administration to obtain procedure privileges in the intensive care unit (ICU). I also shadowed a respiratory therapist and a hospitalist, each for a 40-hour workweek. The remaining 8 months I worked to show how PAs function as a team with physicians to provide better patient care and decrease physician workload, improving their quality of life. Here is a quick inside look of an average week.

Mondays: Sleep Clinic

Consults are scheduled from 8 a.m. to 12 noon. A *consult* is defined as a new patient who is referred from his or her primary physician for an advanced evaluation in the subspecialty of sleep medicine. Each new patient receives an hour of our time. Sleep patients require a very detailed history owing to the various components of sleep hygiene, including temperature, lighting, and television in the bedroom, the bed itself, pets, spouses, and the medical, psychological, and social factors that all affect sleep. All sleep patients require an 8-hour overnight sleep study read by my attending physician, who is board-certified in sleep medicine.

Follow-up appointments are scheduled from 1 p.m. to 5 p.m. These patients have already completed their sleep study and have a specific diagnosis and treatment plan. Obstructive sleep apnea syndrome (OSAS) is the most common sleep disorder and is treated with a continuous positive airway pressure (CPAP) machine. Some of these machines contain a memory card that records the compliance or how many hours per night the patient wears his or her mask. During a follow-up appointment, the card is read and reviewed with the patient to encourage compliance. OSAS strongly correlates with obesity; therefore, the patient is weighed at each visit, and diet and exercise are counseled. Other potential conditions include restless legs syndrome, periodic leg movement disorder, and narcolepsy.

Wednesdays and Fridays: Pulmonary Clinic

Clinic hours are 9 a.m. to 4 p.m., with an hour break for lunch. The three physicians each have a different pulmonary focus. Chronic obstructive pulmonary disease (COPD) and asthma, interstitial lung disease (ILD), and *pulmonary hypertension* subdivide the different clinics.

The COPD and asthma patients all receive aggressive smoking-cessation counseling, observation of proper inhaler usage, and counseling to reduce allergens in the home environment. Many of the ILD patients are referred because of abnormal findings on a *computed tomography (CT)* of the chest, and our job is to investigate the cause. Possibilities include inhaled substances, drugs, connective-tissue disease, and infectious causes. Pulmonary hypertension patients all require a 6-minute walk test at the beginning of their visit to assess exercise capacity. Drug management for this disease is complicated because the patients are often on four different classes of medications. The diagnosis of pulmonary hypertension requires a hospital admission for placement of a *pulmonary artery (PA) catheter* and observation of pulmonary artery pressures while on certain medications to check for a response.

After the medical assistant completes the vital signs and medication list, I am usually the first provider to see the patient. My responsibilities include obtaining a detailed history and performing a physical exam, a review of labs and other results, and answering the patient's questions. I will then give a quick presentation to my attending, and he or she will conclude the visit with additional details. At the end of each clinic day, I will dictate a note for each patient seen that reviews the patient's presentation, the required workup, and the plan designed by my attending physician. This enhances my learning.

Tuesday, Thursday, and Every Third Weekend: Intensive Care Unit and Hospital Work

Sign-out from the partnering night-call physician starts each ICU shift at 6 a.m. Sign-out is a discussion of the patient's progress overnight and a teamwork approach to reviewing pertinent details for the best patient care outcome. I see patients in the ICU one at a time, present to my attending, and then discuss the plan with the nurse. The wide variety of patients makes each day unique.

One patient that will forever stick in my mind is a previously healthy 45-year-old woman who developed a rare and potentially fatal disease 2 weeks after a viral syndrome. Guillain-Barré syndrome is acutely seen and treated in the ICU setting and is a serious disorder in which the body's immune system attacks parts of the nervous system. The patient required ventilator support to breathe in the ICU for 7 days and intravenous high-dose *immunoglobulin* therapy. She was later moved to the medical floor for another 3 weeks, and because of her ongoing diaphragm weakness, she required a *tracheostomy* during her hospital stay. After 3 months of physical therapy, she recovered completely.

Other patients include those with postoperative complications, major *hemoptysis, sepsis* with end-organ damage, interstitial lung disease with pneumonia, and status asthmaticus. During this ICU time, I was able to perform intubations, central and arterial line placements, and *thoracentesis.*

From 1 to 4 p.m., I round on floor patients who required pulmonary or sleep consults. *Rounding* is the act of going to visit your hospitalized patient in his or her room to perform a history and physical exam and to and write out a day-to-day updated treatment plan. It allows the provider to track progress from a clinical and laboratory standpoint. The term *floor patients* is used commonly to describe patients who are residing in a room on the general medical or surgical floor of the hospital and are healthy enough not to require intensive-care support. Patients with severe OSAS, while hospitalized, require bilevel positive airway pressure (BiPAP). With these patients, I will order the machine settings, communicate with the nurse, and encourage patient compliance. Pulmonary consults include pneumonia, asthma or COPD exacerbations, lung cancer, new-onset pulmonary embolus or pulmonary effusion, and chronically ventilated patients. Performing diagnostic and therapeutic thoracentesis on floor patients with pulmonary effusions is also a common task.

During the late afternoons, my attending and I will reround together on the floor patients. While he signs each note, I give a quick presentation, and the attending places any additional orders. The last stop is always the ICU for any nursing updates on patient progress.

I am thankful to have entered this residency immediately after completing PA school because I had the discipline and desire to learn. The key for grasping these subspecialties in 1 year was a commitment to reading during and outside of work. I kept a notepad and took notes about interesting patients and their lab values, diagnostic workups, and treatments. Being the only PA, with pressure to reflect well on the profession, gave me the extra push to study. I have no regrets about completing this residency because it provided a broad knowledge base for my future as a PA. It was this challenge and the fight for PAs in this hospital that propelled me toward PA-student mentoring and this book.

A DAY IN THE LIFE: BARIATRIC MEDICINE

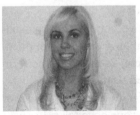

Monika Fuller, PA-C

Coming off my work exit in the morning, I pass by McDonald's, Burger King, Taco Bell, KFC, Dominos, and two Dunkin' Donuts (as if one weren't enough)—all in less than a mile. Mission accomplished: All temptations avoided. The drive every day is a constant reminder of the struggles that we face in fighting the disease known as *obesity*. It is not surprising that over a third of U.S. adults are obese and close to 70 percent are overweight. The obesity epidemic has reached staggering proportions, and the Centers for Disease Control and Prevention (CDC) projects that by 2050, one in three U.S. adults will potentially have diabetes.

My first year of work as a PA is challenging because I decided to specialize in bariatric medicine. Beyond long hours at work, I spend evenings preparing for the exam to become certified in advanced training by the American Board of Bariatric Medicine. After scoring in the top 5 percent of the country, including physicians, I have the confidence I need to practice such a rewarding subspecialty. I learn every day that obesity is a symptom of a chronic medical condition. Although every patient I meet is there to start an aggressive, supervised weight-loss program, each case is certainly unique.

My office is different from most—a PA who acts as the associate medical director owns it. The supervising physician is not present in the office to see patients and only comes in as needed to sign charts. The autonomy of managing my own patients within my scope of practice is very fulfilling.

8:30 a.m.

The day begins by reviewing lab work and finishing charts from the previous night. I check my messages and return a call to a patient who is experiencing nausea while titrating Metformin for newly diagnosed diabetes. I instruct her to keep the medication at 500 mg twice a day and document in the chart to consider Glumetza in the future if side effects persist.

9:00 a.m.

My first patient is a 42-year-old man who started a "protein-sparing modified fast" 1 month ago and has already lost 24 pounds. He presents for his weekly follow-up and is doing well on the diet plan. As a diabetic, he came in taking Actos. Owing to the possible side effects of weight gain and hypoglycemia, I discontinued it and prescribed Metformin at his initial visit. Today he is due for lab tests, so I order a basic metabolic panel (BMP), *hemoglobin A1C*, insulin, and lipid panel. He is without side effects on the new medication, and we discuss the possibility of adding Januvia down the line if we need further glycemic control. I explain that Metformin and Januvia come in combination pill called Janumet and that it controls blood sugar without causing weight gain. Practicing bariatric medicine varies greatly in contrast to my experiences in school. It is not as simple as knowing first-line treatments, and there are many factors to consider, especially when a patient is improving or reversing disease. It is particularly puzzling and frustrating to think that some medications used for diabetes or other comorbidities can induce weight gain, which essentially worsens the disease cycle.

I leave the patient room and glance at the whiteboard, which now has two room numbers listed, signaling that the medical assistant has recorded blood pressure, pulse, and weight and that those patients are ready to be seen. I walk into the next room and begin my consultation with someone who is interested in learning about the weight-loss program. The woman has a *body mass index (BMI)* of 35 and a medical history that includes hypothyroidism, reflux, nonalcoholic fatty liver disease, and osteoarthritis. Her motivation to lose weight stems from wanting to be a good kidney donor for her mother. After further discussion, I tell her that she is a great candidate for the protein-sparing modified fast, and I give her an idea of the diet that she will start at her next appointment. I assure her that we have a successful maintenance program that involves treatment counseling. In addition, I warn her that her underlying medical issues can make losing weight and keeping it off more challenging. Fortunately, as a bariatric medicine specialist, I look beyond the typically searched-for culprit, known as the thyroid. I explore for possible *insulin resistance*, a precursor to diabetes that if left untreated not only will progress to diabetes but also will work against the body and store fat. Then I walk the patient to the front desk, where she sets up an appointment for her initial visit, which will include an electrocardiogram (ECG), lab tests, medical history, and a physical exam. In the subsequent visit, the diet plan will be explained in full detail so that she may begin the 12-week program with weekly visits.

11:00 a.m.

My next patient is new to the office, and her initial visit will take about 1 hour. She is a 51-year-old woman with a BMI of 49.8 and a past medical history of diabetes, hypertension, hyperlipidemia, and obstructive sleep apnea. Her diabetes, at an A1C of 9.8, is poorly controlled on nearly 150 units insulin, including Lantus and Humulog. After completing a medical history, I determine through review of symptoms that she has fatigue and morning headaches and that her husband witnesses snoring and gasping for air. I have clinical suspicion for obstructive sleep apnea, so I fill out a sheet to refer her to a sleep medicine center for further evaluation and possibly a sleep study. Although weight loss helps to treat obstructive sleep apnea (OSA), she might require a continuous positive airway pressure (CPAP) machine. The physical exam is unremarkable except for a velvety hyperpigmented thickening of the skin at the base of the skull not extending to the lateral margins, noted as stage 2 *acanthosis nigricans*. The ECG exhibits normal sinus rhythm, so we begin to review the lab work together. I initiate 4,000 IU/d of vitamin D_3 to treat her vitamin D deficiency, and I also prescribe a potassium supplement that will be needed as replacement while she is on the diet. I review the insulin protocol with the patient, explaining that the insulin must be reduced by half to avoid hypoglycemia because minimal carbohydrates will be consumed. For this reason, and because of its weight-positive properties, I tell her to discontinue Glipizide. I explain that short-term hyperglycemia is safer than hypoglycemia during a protein-sparing modified fast plan. As part of glycemic control, I add an incretin mimetic called Byetta to her Metformin therapy, reviewing directions and possible side effects. I then introduce the patient to our registered nurse (RN), who will detail the diet plan that I've outlined.

There are two notes that have been left on my desk from patients needing refills called into the pharmacy. I then see several routine rechecks with the patients losing 2 to 8 pounds that week and reporting no complaints or side effects. My next patient is a 23-year-old woman with a starting BMI of 38.6 who is in for her 8-week follow-up. She lost 4 pounds this week for a total of 26 pounds. In the initial visit, irregular menstruation was documented with further lab work revealing *polycystic ovarian syndrome*. Her physical exam was positive for acne and *hirsutism*, with labs demonstrating insulin resistance, a principal feature of this endocrine disorder. I started Metformin treatment, and the patient followed up with gynecology to start a contraceptive pill that has helped to regulate her menstrual cycle. Today she needs a refill of Spironolactone, which I started last month to help reduce facial hair growth. As I pull out my prescription pad, she thanks me profusely for the changes that it has made in such a short time not only physically but also with her confidence level.

1:00 p.m.

It is finally lunchtime, so I settle in my office and catch up on several charts that I did not finish in between patients this morning. After writing a letter to a primary physician to update a patient's progress, I eat a healthy lunch and log into my e-mail to read up on my latest medical newsletters. I bookmark a couple of interesting studies to read later tonight and pull up more information on the latest antiobesity medications that were approved by the Food and Drug Administration (FDA) in the past few months. Lorcaserin and Qsymia were the first medications approved in our field in over 13 years, and that validates the growth and value of our specialty.

2:00 p.m.

In the afternoon, I see 15 to 20 patients, and one of them made the 100-pound club! She lost a grand total of 100.5 pounds and is no longer in need of a bilateral knee replacement. By midafternoon, I come across a woman complaining of dizziness for the past few days when standing up. It was seemingly *orthostatic hypotension* secondary to the antihypertensives she was taking, including *diuretics* and *vasodilators*. With a blood pressure (BP) of 110/60 and no significant cardiac history, I instruct the patient to decrease the dose of one of her medications for the next week with the hope of discontinuing the other medications in the coming weeks. She shares that she has been on three blood pressure medications for over 20 years and that she never dreamed of the possibility of stopping them. Fortunately for her, losing over 50 pounds is turning that dream into a reality.

I move on to the patient in the next room, who is a morbidly obese 28-year-old woman who has lost 16 pounds in 4 weeks and is complaining of cravings at night. For the past few weeks we have discussed that *ketosis* curbs hunger, but cravings still may occur. I have counseled her about behavior modification and stress-coping strategies that she has executed in several instances. She has a lot more weight to lose and is doing extremely well. Her ECG shows a normal QTc interval, and there are no contraindications, so to aid with the cravings, I recommend an FDA-approved appetite suppressant that is used by 98 percent of bariatricians. After reviewing directions and side effects, I prescribe Phentermine and tell her to follow up in 1 week.

Similarly, my next patient struggled with cravings the previous few weeks. She is an emotional eater who binges at night. In addition to providing several resources, including referral to a behavioral therapist, I started her on Topamax 25 mg, which has been titrated to 50 mg a day. Since she is taking vitamin C and Tums, as I previously directed, she has not experienced side effects and is feeling more in control.

5:00 p.m.

A woman 5 weeks into the program is waiting in my office, and she is losing weight more slowly than the average, although she is highly motivated and seemingly compliant. With an impaired fasting glucose, A1C of 5.8, triglycerides to high-density lipoprotein (HDL)–cholesterol (TG/HDL) ratio greater than 4, quantitative insulin sensitivity check index (QUICKI) score of 0.35, and a history of gestational diabetes, I suspect insulin resistance. To determine whether I must treat an underlying issue beyond lifestyle intervention, I order a 3-hour glucose tolerance test with insulin. We will follow up next week with results.

One of the following patients is in to review her results from a glucose tolerance test with insulin. The insulin increased from 12 to 90 in the first hour, and the glucose dropped to 52 by the third hour. I diagnose her with hyperinsulinemia with reactive hypoglycemia, and after further education, I provide her with several handouts. I recommend that she continue to lose weight on the diet, but, due to the results, I advise that she begin a medication. We review titration, directions, and side effects, and as she heads to the front desk to make her next appointment, I go to our medicine room to dispense the prescription. For patient convenience, we carry Phentermine, Topamax, and Metformin in our office. I meet her up front with the prescription and encourage her to continue the food diary.

7:00 p.m.

I call two patients who started the diet yesterday to make sure that there are no side effects and that they understand the plan as it was outlined. Since we dispense Class 4 medications in the office, I must do a pill count at the end of each day. As always, the numbers in the book match what is in the cabinet, and I lock the room. Leaving the office, my mind drifts to all the patients whom I have seen today. They inspire me every day to be strong and to make better decisions toward a healthy life. With weekly visits, I quickly become familiar with my patients. As I drive out of the parking lot and into the abyss of temptation, I hope that I have motivated them to keep striving for their goals.

A DAY IN THE LIFE: ENDOCRINE

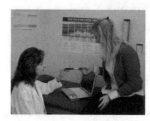

Holly Jodon, MPAS, PA-C

4:45 a.m.

I breathe in the fresh early morning air and soak in the stillness of the predawn hour as I walk into the side entrance of the hospital. As I drink my coffee, I pull up the inpatient list on the computer and check my pager to ensure that all the endocrine consults from the previous night have made it to the list. Next, I review over the last 24 hours to stratify which patients on the floors need to be seen first and record my notes to save time later. This is my week for daily hospital rounds and consultations before going to the office, so I like to get an early start.

5:00 a.m.

The doors to the cardiovascular intensive care unit (CVICU) swing open to hushed yet bustling activity. The sound of monitors and ventilators can be heard as I enter. The night-shift nurses greet me, knowing my presence signals that their shift will be ending soon. They have cared for their patients through the night, so they quickly apprise me of any critical events that have transpired, procedures planned for the day requiring patients to be nothing by mouth (NPO), and patients who may be ready for transfer out of the unit. I review the electronic medical record (EMR) for each patient's status. Most of the patients are postoperative coronary bypass graft (CABG) and/or heart valve surgery and have been started on an intravenous (IV) insulin infusion to control blood sugar, which promotes recovery. Some are known to have type 2 diabetes mellitus (T2DM), some are newly diagnosed as a result of their hospitalization, and some are experiencing transitory postoperative hyperglycemia (high blood sugar), which is the body's compensatory stress response to surgery. My goal this morning is to transition as many patients as possible from their insulin infusions to subcutaneous (injection) insulin and then to oral medications when possible.

Just down from the CVICU, I enter the cardiac care unit. A middle-aged, Middle Eastern woman who immigrated to the United States presented with a cardiac *arrhythmia* due to thyroid storm. We have been monitoring her in the unit while treating her with multiple medications to bring her thyroid hormone levels down. Through an interpreter, she tells me that she is feeling better and is no longer experiencing *palpitations*. I examine her, review her EMR, and discuss her condition over the last 24 hours with her nurse and determine she has stabilized. I write the order to transfer her to the telemetry floor so that we can continue to monitor her as she begins to ambulate and resume activities.

6:00 a.m.

Next, I move to the medical intensive care unit (MICU), where a 23-year-old woman with type 1 diabetes mellitus (T1DM) lies in a coma, intubated and ventilated. She was found unresponsive in her apartment and transported via ambulance to the hospital in diabetic *ketoacidosis* (DKA) from noncompliance and multiple missed insulin dosages. DKA is life-threatening, so correct management is critical and requires a team approach between the pulmonologist/critical-care specialist and endocrine specialist. There is continual monitoring of oxygenation, fluid input and output, blood glucose, and chemistry levels to correct imbalances. Despite our ongoing efforts at diabetic education, counseling, and medical follow-up, this patient remains noncompliant. The patient's family is not present at the moment, so I leave an order requesting a page when they arrive so that we can discuss the severity of potential complications.

A few stations down I see our patient admitted with hyponatremia (low sodium), most likely due to *syndrome of inappropriate antidiuretic hormone (SIADH)*. We are carefully monitoring/regulating IV fluid, electrolyte, and osmolality levels while performing an evaluation to determine the cause in order to correct this condition.

6:45 a.m.

I now transition to see postoperative and interventional cardiac patients. The hall lights are still dimmed, but the nurses' station is lit, and the telemetry technicians are watching a wall of monitors. I sit down at a computer to bring up the records for these patients. The first patients I attend to are those who need their morning dose of insulin changed before breakfast. One patient had blood sugar levels that were dipping down, but he can't remember what he ate the day before, so I find his nurse to inquire if he is eating. She tells me he had some nausea with his pain medication, so I let her know the dosage changes for the morning.

7:00 a.m.

It is change of shift, and the early morning peace gives way to whirlwind of activity. Night-shift nurses are giving reports, while first-shift nurses are taking over their duties. Other providers are rounding on patients, including physicians, PAs, and nurse practitioners, so we share space, computers, and information at the nurses' station.

My next patient is a 62-year-old woman with acute respiratory failure due to an exacerbation of chronic obstructive pulmonary disease (COPD). Her blood sugar levels have been elevated due to high-dose steroids, and she is currently on a tube feeding for nutritional support. She has stabilized enough to be discharged to an extended acute-care facility, so I assess her current condition and confirm the insulin orders to be sent with the patient.

I call my supervising physician to update him on the critical patients who need to be seen and any other concerns I have encountered. We review the list of new consults for the day, which we will see in tandem as a shared hospital visit. He will see the patient, and then write the initial assessment and orders; I will perform a complete history and physical exam and then dictate our entire evaluation for the record.

8:00 a.m.

I move to the pediatric unit, where we have two patients: a 7-year-old girl and an 8-year-old boy, both newly diagnosed with T1DM. These patients and their families must undergo intense education, usually 3 to 5 days, to understand their lifelong requirement for insulin and diabetes management. I assess the parents' and the patients' acceptance of this condition and their confidence in its management.

In the mother-baby unit, I follow up on a patient I saw in the office 3 days ago for her weekly *gestational diabetes mellitus (GDM)* visit. When she told me that her blood sugar levels were "good" even though she was "not taking her insulin," I called her obstetrician's office to have her evaluated emergently. She subsequently underwent a cesarean section that day for placental regression and delivered a healthy baby boy. Currently, her blood sugar levels are normal postpartum, so she will need to follow up with a glucose tolerance test in our office in 6 weeks.

9:00 a.m.

Next, I head to the *dialysis* unit, where patients with kidney failure are undergoing treatment, most in recliners, but a few in beds. I hear the constant hum of the machines that clear their bloodstream through a surgically placed IV port. They undergo dialysis three times per week as outpatients, so this remains their routine unless they receive a kidney transplant.

10:00 a.m.

My next endocrine consult is to assess the residual pituitary function of a 45-year-old man who has had a pituitary tumor resected. I order blood hormone levels and review the preliminary chemistry values.

The next consult, a 52-year-old woman, is a postoperative thyroidectomy patient by the otolaryngologist for a cancerous nodule we found in the office earlier this month. Our endocrine role is to monitor for abnormal calcium levels, replace her thyroid hormone, and talk about follow-up for further treatment of the thyroid cancer.

11:00 a.m.

I follow up on our remaining patients on the medical and surgical floors and then head back to the office for lunch.

1:00 p.m.

I now begin my afternoon in the office. Diabetes, especially T2DM, is rising to epidemic proportions in our country, reflected in the number of patients referred to our office for management of uncontrolled disease and complications. This afternoon I see a patient with newly diagnosed GDM who needs to begin insulin for the safety of her unborn child. I see a 58-year-old man whose T2DM is uncontrolled on oral medications, so we discuss adding an injectable incretin mimetic. A 64-year-old man, disabled due to complications of *neuropathy* and foot ulcers, presents postoperatively after amputation of his right forefoot. I adjust his insulin to control blood sugar, which will maximize his wound healing and overall health.

Next, a 76-year-old woman is here for follow-up of osteoporosis, including her annual *dexa scan* and renewal of her medications. Her scan shows further loss of bone mass even though she is compliant with her oral therapy. We talk about a once-a-year IV option for treatment of osteoporosis and schedule the needed blood work prior to an infusion appointment.

3:00 p.m.

In the next exam room, a 32-year-old man with T1DM is currently using an *insulin pump* and a blood glucose sensor that provides continuous tissue/blood sugar monitoring. The use of both these technologies allows for a better understanding of insulin infusion and corresponding blood sugar trends over a 24-hour basis. We are able to map out the time of day he is having low blood sugar levels and reprogram his insulin pump accordingly.

A 38-year-old woman presents for follow-up of *Hashimoto's hypothyroidism*. I increased her dose of thyroid replacement at her last visit, and she tells me that she is feeling better. Her fatigue is gone, her energy level is better, and she is no longer constipated. Clinically, her exam is normal, and her current thyroid blood level results are normal. I give her the prescription for the new dose with plans to follow up in 6 months unless her symptoms recur.

Next, I see a 26-year-old African-American woman who was referred for infertility problems. Her lab results confirm she has congenital adrenal hyperplasia (CAH), but her physical exam and age at presentation indicate that she has a mild case. In order for her to conceive, hormone levels will need to be normalized, so we discuss how this will occur.

In the next room I see a 41-year-old woman who underwent an ultrasound-guided fine-needle aspiration of a thyroid nodule in our office a week ago. I give her the good news that the pathology was *benign* and that we will monitor this with periodic ultrasounds to ensure that it does not change in size or density.

My last patient of the day is a 14-year-old boy who is seen for short stature, currently being treated with human growth hormone. He was making great progress on his height, but today's measurement is the same as the previous one. His mother tells me that he has been reluctant to adhere to the injections, and he tells me, "I just don't care that I'm shorter than everyone else. I get teased at school no matter what." We discuss that this is the only time we will be able to increase his height because as he matures his bones fuse and his height will remain the same into adulthood. We talk about ways he can cope, and he is agreeable to continue the therapy for another 6 months.

5:00 p.m.

After I finish with patients, I take time to address phone messages, call-backs, review lab results, and refill prescriptions.

5:30 p.m.

If any more consults come in for the day, I will head back to the hospital to see those patients.

In our office, the PAs alternate hospital weeks, so the more PAs employed, the less often we cover the hospital. We work under the supervision of an adult endocrinologist and a pediatric endocrinologist, so we see patients of all ages and cases that intersect all areas of medicine: critical care, cardiology, pulmonary, gastroenterology, obstetrics, otolaryngology, oncology, general surgery, neurosurgery, cardiovascular surgery, neurology/rehabilitative, and psychiatric. The patients admitted to the hospital are dealing with life-altering conditions that in many cases can be life-threatening. Our office patients require ongoing follow-up for preventative care to achieve and maintain health. It takes a concerted effort to educate patients and motivate them to control this disease, but with so many new medications and more insulin options available than ever before, this is an exciting time in endocrine care.

Holly Jodon is an Endocrine PA at Metabolic Disease Associates, Inc., in Erie, PA. The author has indicated no relationships to disclose relating to the content of this piece.

A DAY IN THE LIFE: CARDIOTHORACIC SURGERY

Jonathan E. Sobel, PA-C, FAPACVS, MBA

Walking from the parking garage to the hospital, I am amazed by the stark contrast between the serene parklike grounds of the hospital set among the chaotic rush of several thousand staff members moving toward the entrance of what equates to a small city. I hear the soothing sounds of our resident birds saying good morning from their perches in our bamboo garden, the rush of our waterfall fountain in chorus with the chirping. I dodge around the cars pulling into the front circle as I wonder what my day brings and when I will find myself saying goodnight to the aviary on my way home.

6:30 a.m.

Dropping off my bag and donning my lab coat, I make a run up to the cardiothoracic intensive care unit (CTICU). I check in with the night coverage team to see how our patients from yesterday have done. One patient was completing weaning trials and would be extubated shortly. Everyone else was already weaned and sitting upright in a chair. They will have their chest tubes removed after rounds and go on their first walking expedition with their freshly repaired hearts.

6:45 a.m.

I print a census list and run off to the operating room (OR) to check the schedule for any last-minute changes. Grabbing a pair of scrubs from the vending machine, I meet the rest of the OR team to go over the room assignments for today's cases. Surgeon and team preferences, training needs, case requirements, and on-call schedules go into the decision, and shortly everyone has the day tentatively mapped.

7:00 a.m.

After a quick change into scrubs, I join the interdisciplinary team gathering in the conference room for morning rounds. The patients are presented, the chest x-rays (CXRs) reviewed, and the plan of care for each patient decided. The value of having our nurses, surgeons, therapists, social workers, physician assistants (PAs), and intensivists all on the same page cannot be overstated.

7:30 a.m.

I help the team place our patient on the table for a coronary artery bypass graft (CABG) and aortic valve replacement. I place an arterial line while reassuring the patient that he will be in the best of hands with the care team he has chosen. I assist the anesthesiologist with the airway and then quickly reach for my ultrasound machine. Evaluating both saphenous veins from ankle to groin, I find that the right vein is of suitable caliber without varicosities or *thrombosis* and carefully mark the course of the vein. I am able to tell the surgeon with confidence that there will be suitable conduit for the case. I check my *endoscopic* equipment after inserting the Foley catheter and positioning the patient; now it's time to scrub.

8:00 a.m.

I harvest and prepare two segments of vein while the surgeon takes down the left internal thoracic artery. Owning the vein harvest from skin to skin, an operation within the operation, I am keenly aware of the great responsibility and thankful that I have chosen to work in a specialty that affords such autonomy. Later, I take my place across the table from the surgeon, and we put the patient on *cardiopulmonary bypass* through cannulas the size of garden hoses. Diverting the blood in this manner, we give the heart its first rest in 78 years while we perform our work. My harvested veins become grafts sewn to reroute oxygen-rich blood past diseased coronary arteries, and an aortic valve immobile with cauliflower-like calcium is carefully exchanged for one made of bovine *pericardium*. We slide the new valve down parachute sutures of alternating blue and white and work swiftly to tie each knot down tight. Suture lines checked multiple times, we remove the patient from the pump and begin our closure routine.

12:00 Noon

I transport our patient to the CTICU, handing over his care to my colleagues in the unit while we settle him in. I go out to the waiting room to let his wife and son know that they are able to visit for a short while. I try to prepare them for the sight of ventilators, chest tubes with bloody tubing, and multiple protruding catheters from their unconscious husband and father. Signs of concerned relief are palpable and are offset by gentle reminders that the first 48 hours are considered critical.

12:20 p.m.

I grab a bite at my desk while returning calls and e-mails. Then I head back to the OR to break a colleague out from a long case. When she returns, I close up the open leg incision before breaking scrub.

2:00 p.m.

I hurry back to the conference room in time for our departmental quality meeting. The focus is on a recent bump in our sternal wound infection rates. We discuss the offending organisms, our preparation and drape routine to make the field sterile, our antibiotic choices, and a myriad of other factors before deciding on a course of action.

3:00 p.m.

I return to the CTICU to see that my patient has wakened a bit and moved all four extremities, although not yet to command. After *debridement* of such a calcified valve, we are always concerned with *embolic* events, and I am encouraged by this report. Urine output has been brisk, hemodynamic parameters excellent, and chest tube drainage minimal.

3:30 p.m.

I head back to the OR and take over assisting a second case that a colleague had started earlier. I am the late guy and on call tonight, and thus I will repeat this action until all cases are done and settled.

7:00 p.m.

I drop off the last patient to the CTICU, but I am having trouble finding the night coverage team. While I settle the patient in, a nurse tells me that they are down in the emergency room (ER) evaluating what sounds like an acute type A *aortic dissection*. I call home and give my wife the all too familiar news and realize that the birds will have to wait to say goodbye.

A DAY IN THE LIFE: OCCUPATIONAL MEDICINE AND URGENT CARE

Patrick F. Freeman, MHA, MMS, PA-C

I work in occupational medicine and urgent care. For the most part, my day consists of treating work-related injuries and illnesses. Many are orthopedic in nature, but psychology, neurology, head, ears, eyes, nose, and throat (HEENT), pulmonology, and infectious diseases are also frequently addressed in my practice. In occupational medicine, the goal is to get the injured worker back to his or her previous level of function and returned to work as soon as possible. I eschew a sedentary recovery for one that actively integrates therapy and maximal work function, even if it means a patient is performing very simple and light-intensity work initially. Studies have shown that the longer an employee is out of work due to an injury, the more likely it is that he or she will never return to any type of work.

My day begins at 7 a.m. I arrive at the clinic 10 minutes before my shift starts to find the parking lot full and six or seven young men waiting outside the main entrance. This is a typical sight because most people want to get their various physical exams and drug screens done early so that they do not miss any work. Most of the men have their hands filled with coffee cups, and one has a large can of a popular energy drink he has just finished. Two of these men will be my first patients of the day.

Before I start seeing patients, I review my schedule for the day. I have 15 patients scheduled today, and many of their names are familiar. However, they only represent a portion of my work for the day. I also may see just as many walk-in patients today. I sit down and go over the few charts that require my review and sign off on lab results and specialist consultations.

7:05 a.m.

One of the young men I walked past just minutes earlier had twisted his ankle at a construction site the day before. He is limping, and when he pulls off his work boot, I am greeted with a swollen, purple ankle. He is able to move it some, but it hurts. Sensation to light touch is intact, and pulses are normal. His heart rate and blood pressure are both elevated. I talk to him briefly about his caffeine consumption and proper nutrition. Despite his ability to walk on the ankle, I get an x-ray to rule out a fracture. As expected, the x-ray comes back negative for bony injury. I recommend nonsteroidal anti-inflammatory drugs (NSAIDs), and I prescribe a walking boot and refer him to physical therapy. I also place him on work restrictions to prevent further injury to ankle and to prevent any other injury due to his decreased mobility and agility. I encourage him to quit smoking and cite studies that show that smoking delays recovery from musculoskeletal injuries. After I escort him to the checkout area, I contact his employer to notify him of the patient's work restrictions.

7:20 a.m.

Several truck drivers have come in for their department of transportation (DOT) physicals. Two go without a hitch, but the third requires further follow-up. He is in his fifties, snores loudly per his report, is overweight with hypertension, a Mallampati score of 3, and neck circumference of 19 inches. These are all signs of sleep apnea, so he will need a sleep study before he can be certified to drive. Mallampati is a scoring classification determined by looking inside the mouth. Visibility of only the soft and hard palates and base of the uvula is a class 3.

8:00 a.m.

I see a few patients for reevaluation of their injuries. One patient with a healed scalp laceration has his staples removed and is placed at maximum medical improvement and discharged. A young woman with a concussion sustained when a box of automotive parts fell onto her head from a height of 9 feet at work is progressing, albeit slowly. I review her chart and the specialist's notes. She is suffering from postconcussive syndrome with headaches and occasional vertigo. I decide to keep her off work and advise her not to drive as long as these symptoms continue. She will start vestibular therapy and continue her medications for headaches. I see a few more patients for DOT physicals, and they are all deemed fit for duty.

10:30 a.m.

Five injury rechecks have come and gone, all progressing as expected. The sixth is a young man who was struck by a car in a parking lot at his work site. He is suffering with significant muscular guarding in his neck and back, a sizable hematoma to the back of his head, and several abrasions on his arms and back. While all of his x-rays and computed tomographic (CT) scans have come back normal, his muscles remain in a state of stiffness and spasm. I walk him to physical therapy and adjust his medications to curtail the sedation and dizziness he is experiencing from the narcotic pain medications prescribed in the emergency room the night before. I keep him off work due to his continued sedation, dizziness, and inability to stand up straight or bend at the waist without significant discomfort.

11:00 a.m.

A young woman returns for a recheck on the progress of a *corneal abrasion* she sustained when a coworker accidentally struck her in the eye with a sheet of paperboard. She has no complaints of discomfort or discharge from the eye. I instill fluorescein dye into her eye and inspect it with a *slit lamp*. The abrasion has healed, and I discharge her from care. I work through respiratory physicals for two young men who will start work for an asbestos abatement company. Their chest x-rays are clear, and the their pulmonary function tests and physical exams are normal. A few phone calls to employers and I am off to lunch.

12:00 Noon

A young man presents for urgent care complaining of right ear pain. He has had a head cold and has been congested for 3 days. I look into his right ear and find a ruptured *tympanic membrane* and a small amount of blood. After many prompts, he tells me that he had used a cotton swab to clean his ear not long before the ear pain began. He has apparently ruptured the tympanic membrane with the cotton swab. I assure him that these typically heal on their own but that there is nothing I can do for it now. I prescribe him ibuprofen 600 mg for the pain and refer him to an ear, nose, and throat specialist for follow-up.

1:00 p.m.

Three rechecks are in, all for back pain, all sustained after improperly lifting heavy objects or people. These three are all in physical therapy, on restricted duty, and taking NSAIDs. As one nears discharge, I review with her the proper way to lift and to avoid reaching or twisting while lifting and to ask for help whenever needed. The other two are weeks from discharge but are improving daily. I talk to the physical therapist about their status and progress.

2:00 p.m.

The last of my scheduled patients comes in. He is a certified nursing assistant who 3 weeks ago tore his rotator cuff trying to catch an elderly patient who had started to roll out of bed. His magnetic resonance imaging (MRI) confirms fully detached supraspinatous and infraspinatous tendons. He is attending physical therapy regularly and regaining some movement in the shoulder while he awaits surgery to repair his shoulder. Despite his pain, he is working light duty and takes only over-the-counter medication for his pain. He is clearly motivated, and I feel confident that his outcome will be good.

3:00 to 5:00 p.m.

I catch up on charts while I await the afternoon rush of new injuries that is particular to my clinic. I contact an employer regarding the circumstances of a patient I treated the evening before. After donating blood at her work, she returned to her desk only to pass out. She struck her head on the desk and sustained a large hematoma to her forehead. After confirming the details, I call the patient to inform her that her injury, while sustained at work, is not work-related and that she should follow up with her primary-care provider for further care.

A young woman comes in for a burn sustained to her left hand while preparing food at a fast-food restaurant and a man in his forties comes in shortly thereafter for a 7-cm laceration sustained to his middle finger while taking out the trash. The woman's burn is superficial and will do fine with burn cream and bandaging for next few days. The man's laceration is deep but thankfully does not involve the flexor or extensor tendons. After getting the bleeding under control, I place two deep absorbable sutures and close with several simple interrupted sutures. His wound is dressed, and my final patient of the day leaves at 15 minutes after 5:00.

Before I leave for the day, I check on outstanding dictations and incomplete charts. It is 5:30, no one is waiting outside the doors, and the parking lot is empty.

Reflecting on the day, I feel good that I was able to return several people to work, allowing them to earn a living and support their families as well as maintain their sense of worth and personal identity. I was also able to ensure that several prospective employees were fit for duty and able to safely perform their respective work duties. A solid economy is based on the workforce, and I return home feeling that I have made my contribution to keep the cogs of industry moving.

A DAY IN THE LIFE: PLASTIC SURGERY

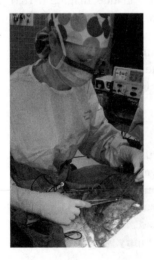

Kristina Peterson Marsack, MS, PA-C

I have been a physician assistant (PA) in plastic surgery at Ben Taub General Hospital (BTGH) for over 7 years. Ben Taub is a level I trauma center and county hospital in the Texas Medical Center in Houston. I work with several attending plastic surgeons who have an assigned day of the week to oversee our cases and two plastic surgery physician residents who rotate on the service for 4 months at a time. The daily change in attendings and the constant flux of residents allow me to be the primary point of contact for the hospital staff and the continuity of care for patients. This position requires surgical and clinical skills, leadership qualities, organization, good people skills and an ability to be the glue that holds together the needs of the patients, nurses, and physicians.

Every day is different depending on the operating room (OR) and clinic schedules; here is an example of a possible Wednesday.

7:00 a.m.

The day starts with team rounds in the critical wound unit (CWU) with the chief of BTGH plastic surgery and the current residents. We discuss each patient's hospital course, operative plan, and discharge needs before dividing up the patient care and charting needs.

7:30 a.m.

On returning to the office, I review the OR schedule with the team and make changes to accommodate the new trauma patients who were admitted overnight. In order to maximize future OR time, I contact a few elective patients to schedule their surgery dates.

8:00 a.m.

As the surgeons start a delayed unilateral breast reconstruction case using an abdominal free flap (transverse rectus abdominis myocutaneous, or TRAM flap) in the OR, I see postoperative patients and perform minor surgeries in the plastics clinic. I also work with the hospital staff to get the next day's OR cases posted.

8:15 a.m.

My first patient returns today for her first expansion of her right breast tissue expander, which was placed 3 weeks ago at the time of her mastectomy. She is feeling well but is nervous to start the expansion process. I reassure her that her discomfort will be limited to a prick of a needle and a few days of muscle soreness. She asks her husband to hold her hand. I locate the port with the port finder, clean the area with Betadine, and begin infusing injectable saline into the expander. She tolerates 60 cc of fluid without difficulty. She lets out a big sigh of relief when I finish the infusion and states that it wasn't too bad. She will return for the same process in 1 week.

8:30 a.m.

In the next room, a 47-year-old woman returns for her first postoperative visit after a left immediate TRAM flap reconstruction performed 2 weeks ago. She states that she is happy with her results and is hoping that I can remove all her drains today. Her breast flap is warm, pink, and viable with good contour. Her incisions are healing well. Her abdomen has a viable umbilicus, and there is no sign of hernia or wound dehiscence. Her breast drain is putting out less than 20 cc daily of serosanguineous fluid, a thin and red discharge composed of serum and blood. This means that the drain is ready for removal; however, her abdominal drains are still draining excessively and will remain in place for another week. I make sure that she has enough antibiotics and let her know that her pathology shows negative margins of ductal carcinoma in situ (DCIS). I then verify that she has her breast surgery and oncology follow-up appointments.

8:55 a.m.

As I leave the room, I receive a page from my clinical case manager to discuss social issues related to the patient in CWU bed 8. He needs a wheelchair, so I sign into the computer and complete the order.

9:00 a.m.

Then I walk into the third patient's room, a postoperative check after a wide local excision of a basal cell carcinoma on his nasal ala that required a nasolabial flap. First, I give him the good news that his final pathology margins are clear. Then, after examining his wounds, I remove his sutures and discuss the plan for division and inset of his flap in a second surgery 2 weeks from now.

9:10 a.m.

The next patient is here for her final breast tissue expansion. After expansion, we discuss her next surgery for implant exchange with silicone implants. I take measurements and pictures to help plan for the surgery and then schedule her for our preoperative screening clinic (POSC) in 4 to 6 weeks.

9:30 a.m.

A 32-year-old breast reduction patient presents on postoperative day (POD) 6. She has been wearing her surgical bra and has been compliant with her wound care, but she complains of some wound breakdown. On inspection, she has a 3- × 3-cm wound at the trifurcation point near her inframammary fold. There is good granulation tissue and no pus or cellulitis. The patient denies any fever or other signs of infection. I instruct her on wet-to-dry Kerlix dressing changes. Her Jackson Pratt (JP) drains, one for each breast, had less than 20 cc of serosanguineous fluid per day, so I remove them. The patient is advised to stop her antibiotics and return to clinic in 2 weeks for reassessment.

9:45 a.m.

I receive a page from the POSC clinic because a preoperative patient wants to change her surgery date. I take the patient's information and let the nurse know that I will contact her later.

9:50 a.m.

Returning my focus to my clinic, I enter the exam room to see a 19-year-old woman who is status post left axillary latissimus dorsi myocutaneous flap reconstruction for *hidradenitis* suppurativa. She states that she is feeling well but that there has been a lot of drainage from around her flap. She denies fever, chills, nausea, and vomiting. On examination, she has a viable flap, but there is an area medially that has purulent drainage, concerning for hidradenitis recurrence. Since the area is small, I instruct her on local wound care with wet-to-dry Kerlix dressings and prescribe antibiotics. The patient is scheduled for follow-up in 2 weeks.

10:15 a.m.

Another postoperative breast tissue expander patient presents on POD 7. She complains of right breast pain without warmth or fever. On exam, she has an intact incision but a very tender, mildly erythematous breast, concerning for seroma versus infection. Her tissue expander is palpable with some overlying fluctuance. Her JP drain is putting out 65 cc per day of murky fluid, which I send for aerobic and anaerobic cultures. I contact my supervising physician to inform him of her condition. While I wait for him to come see her, I proceed to get her history and physical exam and admission orders together. Once we see her together, we decide to consult interventional radiology to place a *percutaneous* drain in order to attempt to salvage the implant. The patient is given instructions for admission.

10:45 a.m.

A patient status post open reduction and internal fixation of a right angle of mandible and mandbulomaxillary fixation (MMF) of left subcondylar fractures returns to clinic for his 2-week follow-up. I order and review his Panorex. His arch bars, MMF, and plates are intact, and his fracture is in good alignment. The patient reports feeling well with numbness in the right mental nerve distribution. I counsel him on typical resolution of sensation within 3 months. He is also asking to eat more than a full liquid diet. Since his intraoral incisions are intact, he has good occlusion, and there is no evidence of infection, I cut his MMF wires out and place him in elastics. I explain how to use the elastics and that they are important for training his jaw to close properly as his subcondylar fracture heals. I remind him that he is to follow a strict nonchew diet and to have good oral hygeine. He is scheduled for follow-up in 1 month.

11:00 a.m.

Two weeks ago I performed nipple reconstruction on a breast reconstruction patient; today, she presents for follow-up. She previously had a right TRAM flap breast reconstruction, and a portion of the TRAM skin was elevated and folded on itself to create a nipple mound. She has been using a nipple protector and Bacitracin since the procedure. I remove the protector and examine the small flaps to ensure their viability and then remove the sutures. She looks great, but I remind her that the nipples frequently flatten once she starts wearing tight clothing or sleeping on her stomach. I recommend using the protector for as long as she will tolerate it. She is then scheduled for a follow-up procedure in 3 months for nipple tattooing.

11:25 a.m.

Finally, my last patient in clinic is here for minor surgery to excise a potentially malignant 4-mm lesion on the forehead. I find a Spanish interpreter to help me acquire informed consent from the patient for the procedure. I then perform the timeout, use a marking pen to circumscribe the lesion with 1-mm margins in order to optimize complete excision, and then inject the area with 1% lidocaine with epinepherine. As the nurse preps the patient, I scrub and gown. I double-check to make sure that the patient is insensate, and I begin to excise the lesion with a no. 15 blade down to subcutaneous fat, using needle-tip Bovie *cautery* for hemostasis. I mark the specimen with a silk suture for orientation (12:00 short stitch, 9:00 long stitch) and place it in the specimen cup held by the nurse. Using tenotomy scissors, I undermine the skin flaps a few centimeters to decrease tension. I place a deep dermal 4-0 Monocryl suture in the center of the wound and then evaluate and excise the lateral dog-ears. Fortunately, the lesion was along a rhytid (or forehead wrinkle), and the scar is able to be placed within the crease. I finish the deep dermals and complete the closure with a 5-0 running subcutaneous Monocryl suture. The area is cleaned with normal saline, and Steri-Strips are placed. I then scrub out, wash up, and write the procedure note with follow-up next Friday to ensure that final pathology will be complete. The patient is counseled regarding the need for further surgery if the lesion is malignant and the margins are positive for residual tumor.

12:30 p.m.

I finish my charting in clinic, grab some lunch, and head to the plastics office. On the way, I get stopped by a nurse to advance a patient's diet, change his pain medications, and reorder Metoprolol. While I eat, I update the OR wait list, make some changes to the OR schedule, and add the clinic pictures taken earlier in the day to our database.

2:00 p.m.

I receive a page from the OR letting me know that the surgeons are ready for me to close the patient's donor site for the TRAM breast reconstruction. I proceed to scrub in while the surgeons are performing the *microanastamosis* of the deep inferior epigastric artery to the internal mammary vessels in order to reestablish blood flow to the abdominal tissue that is now on the patient's chest to create a new breast mound.

First, I finish elevating the abdominal flap in a bell shape along the rib line to the xyphoid. Then I irrigate the abdomen thoroughly and ensure good hemostasis. Using 4-0 Vicryl sutures, I loosely reapproximate the rectus muscle. Then the fascia is closed primarily with 0 Ethibond interrupted buried figure-of-eight sutures to prevent hernia or bulging of the abdominal contents. Two JP drains are placed to allow for serosanguineous output from the wound. The abdominal wound edges are then approximated with skin staples. The location of the umbilicus is identified, and an incision is made to begin the inset. The umbilical skin edges are closed, and Xeroform gauze is placed in the neoumbilicus.

Focus then turns to the long abdominal incision. Bilateral dog-ears (excess tissue at the lateral edges of the incision) are marked and excised with a no. 10 blade and Bovie cautery. Scarpas *fascia* and the dermis are closed, and Dermabond is used to cover the incision.

The surgeons have finished the microsurgery and are insetting the flap to create the new breast. I scrub out to take pictures of the patient's on-table results. After the anesthesiologist extubates the patient, I assist the surgeons in moving the patient to the stretcher and transporting her to the post-anesthesia care unit (PACU). My team then reconvenes in the office to discuss any new patient-care issues.

5:00 p.m.

I gather my bags and walk back to the parking garage, mentally recounting my day. In surgery, you work hard until the work is done and then you go home. The amazing thing about life as a surgical PA is that no two days are ever the same. Plans change, at any moment an emergency case can roll through the door, and your initial schedule is thrown out the window. My favorite part of being a surgical PA is that we are truly team members; everyone on my service feels ownership in each patient's care, and we have a shared goal to make that person better. And finally, the best part of being in plastic surgery is that the results are visible (in most cases) and usually very instantaneously gratifying.

A DAY IN THE LIFE: PEDIATRICS

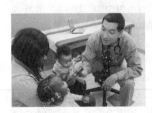

Chris Barry, PA-C, MMSc

When I entered physician assistant (PA) school, I came in with an open mind about my future field of practice. I had originally leaned toward family medicine or emergency medicine. However, I developed a liking for pediatrics right from the start of my clinical rotations. Pediatrics was my very first rotation, and I started out a little nervous working with small children. As I observed my preceptor and started seeing my own patients, I became comfortable with children of all ages in short order. I remember one day toward the end of my rotation, a parent of an infant told me after I saw her child, "Some people choose their work; some are called. You were called." I thanked her, initially not understanding her statement, but then realizing, "Wow, I *am* a perfect fit for pediatrics. This is my calling." As long as I can remember, I have always been a "kid magnet." I think the fact that I am 6 feet 5 inches tall makes children intrigued by my height. I am a big kid at heart, and I love to relate to children on their level, literally and figuratively. After that initial pediatrics rotation, I chose to do two elective rotations in outpatient pediatrics and one in the pediatric emergency department.

After graduating from the Emory University PA Program in 2000, I found a great job in general pediatrics in an Atlanta suburb. Dr. Jeffrey Cooper was my employer, and I learned a lot about pediatrics from him and my two nurse-practitioner coworkers. I really enjoyed watching my patients grow and getting to know their families. After 5 years working with Dr. Cooper, I made the tough decision to move back to North Carolina. My wife and I wanted to be closer to our families after the birth of our first child, Jessica. For the past 6 years, I have worked for a large pediatric practice in Raleigh, NC, during which time we had another daughter, Leah. I have also taken on several volunteer positions related to my profession, some of which I will discuss in this piece.

7:15 a.m.

After conferring by phone with my physician colleague, I arrive at a local hospital to make newborn rounds. My colleague will be rounding at a different hospital this morning (we make rounds at three area hospitals). Rounds involve examination of newborn babies to assess their overall health. This can be challenging because we often have several babies to see and must finish in time to return to the office to see patients there. Luckily, today there are only three babies for me to see, and they all appear pretty straightforward. The first two babies go well—no major findings, feeding well, no issues with jaundice, and minimal weight loss. When I arrive in the room of the third baby, I find both parents happily lying in the hospital bed with their newborn son on top of them. I find out that the baby is breast-feeding well and seems to be voiding and stooling well. His weight loss is about 5 percent, which is normal, and he is due to be circumcised today. In our area, the obstetric (OB) physicians perform circumcisions, whereas in other parts of the country the pediatric providers perform the circumcisions. I examine the baby and note that the exam is normal, except for two toes on his right foot that appear to be webbed together by a fairly thin flap of skin. The parents have noticed this, they say, and ask if the OB could just clip that because he would be cutting their baby's foreskin anyway. I explain to them that the OB is only qualified to perform circumcisions and will refer their son to a different specialist as an outpatient. The parents are okay with this explanation. I complete the chart and scuttle to our satellite office in Clayton, southeast of Raleigh.

8:30 a.m.

I arrive at our Clayton office ready to give my presentation on adolescent immunizations to the nurses. About once a month, one of the providers presents a clinically relevant topic to our nursing staff either before office hours or during lunch. I chose to talk about vaccines because I have fielded several questions recently from nurses about the need for certain vaccines in our adolescent patients. Fortunately, I had just given a talk at the American Academy of Physician Assistants (AAPA) annual conference on this subject. There are about 15 nurses in our conference room, and we are linked up electronically to our practice's four other offices. I am proud to talk about the importance and benefits of vaccines. Because the nurses are the first point of contact for our patients, it is important that they are comfortable making strong vaccine recommendations. We are all a team, and our goal is healthy children. I keep this phrase in mind throughout the day and repeat it inside my head when I face a particularly difficult challenge.

9:20 a.m.

My first patient of the day is a 17-year-old boy here for his annual exam. In reviewing his chart, I remember that he had auditory hallucinations, anxiety, and depression at last year's annual exam, for which I referred him to psychiatry. I did not see a scanned note from a psychiatrist in his chart, so I will ask him if he ever went.

When I walk in the exam room, he is sitting on the exam table, well kempt and alert. I strike up a conversation about his summer plans, how school went last year, and how things are going in general. I always like to break the ice before beginning the physical exam and discussing any serious subjects. He mentions that he likes music, plays the guitar, and does some music production at home. We find common ground in music, and I give him a sample of my rapping skills, in case he had any doubts! I think this put him at ease because he nodded to my rap. His physical exam is normal, and I excuse Mom from the room during the exam for my patient's privacy.

While mom is out of the room, I delve a little further into his previous mental health problems. It turns out a lot of his problems were related to a lack of sleep, a common problem with busy teenagers. Last year I had recommended taking all electronic devices, including the television and video game system out of his room. In addition, I recommended charging his cell phone in a separate room overnight so that he would not be tempted to use his phone for texting or the Internet while he should be sleeping. He took my advice to heart and now gets between 8 and 9 hours of sleep every night. He reports that he never went to the psychiatrist because once he fixed his sleep hygiene, his hallucinations, anxiety, and depression got better. I was happy to hear such a successful outcome and congratulated him on this. Of course, I told him if things change and he needs to see a psychiatrist, I would help him make that appointment. His physical exam was normal, and I signed his sports physical form, happy to see him healthy, both mentally and physically.

10:45 a.m.

A seeming busload of patients checks in on my schedule simultaneously. Fortunately, between the excellent nurses I work with and my helpful colleagues, I am able to see all the patients with a minimum wait time. This morning I see a lot of children with coughs, fevers, sore throats, and ear infections—the "bread and butter" of pediatrics. I see a classic case of strep throat and wish I had a student working with me today to see it. I often train PA students from my alma mater, Emory University, as well as medical students from the University of North Carolina. I will always be grateful for my clinical preceptors who taught me so much in PA school. Volunteering as a clinical preceptor allows me to give back to my profession, and it keeps me sharp. To have to explain how and why I do things the way I do forces me to go back and look up guidelines and recommendations and to come up with a good differential diagnosis list in my mind.

12:30 p.m.

Lunch time! This will be a working lunch. We don't have an office meeting today, but I have two calls to make during lunch, related to my volunteer activities with the PA profession. The first is a conference call with the new American Academy of Physician Assistants (AAPA) CEO, Jenna Dorn, to discuss the academy's strategic plans and how they are going to implement them. This is a conference call with all 21 of the medical liaisons within the AAPA. Medical liaisons serve as conduits of information between AAPA and the respective physician organizations and are the public face of our profession to our respective organizations. This is my fifth year serving as the AAPA medical liaison to the American Academy of Pediatrics (AAP). It is an honor to serve in this role, and it's a great feeling to represent my fellow PAs in dealings with the leaders of the AAP. The AAP is a wonderful organization with a similar mission to that of the AAPA, and that is to provide high-quality health care for our patients. After a great call with the AAPA, I make a quick call to the AAP's director of strategic planning to iron out plans for implementation of PA membership to the AAP. Thanks largely to the work of the AAP liaisons before me, PAs are now able to join the AAP as national affiliate members. I feel that our partnership with the AAP will show pediatricians that we share their goals and work in conjunction with them to form a healthcare team.

1:30 p.m.

Back to work seeing patients. A baby girl is here for her 2-month well-child visit. Not only do I enjoy seeing the babies, but I love to see the excitement on the new parents' faces. I review the developmental screening information the parents had completed the day before online, and everything looks good. For a baby's well-child visit, not only do I examine the baby physically, but I check the baby's development and growth provide nutritional and parenting advice, respond to parents' questions, and update the baby's immunizations. The nurse tells me that the parents have concerns with the pertussis vaccine because the baby's father had a serious reaction to the pertussis vaccine when he was a child, about 25 years ago. When dealing with vaccine-hesitant parents, I never know how the vaccine discussion will go, but I always present the information the same way, objectively and scientifically, allowing the parents to make the best choice for their infant.

As I conduct my exam, I notice that the baby is growing well and has increased in length, weight, and head circumference since the last visit. I answer the parents' questions on feeding and sleep, and then we begin to discuss immunizations. Mom wants to give the DTaP vaccine separately from the others and come back in 1 to 2 weeks for the other vaccines. I explain to them that although I will do whatever they like, I recommend giving all the recommended vaccines today. I explain that the pertussis vaccine used today is far different from the pertussis vaccine from 25 years ago. The whole-cell pertussis vaccine that caused so many fevers and persistent crying is no longer used. Instead, an acellular pertussis vaccine with a thousand-fold fewer antigens is used, causing much fewer side effects. Dad says that he is fine going either way, and we discuss the risks of delaying vaccination. Ultimately, I present the scientific evidence on the safety and efficacy of the vaccines and tell them that I vaccinated both my girls according to the Centers for Disease Control and Prevention (CDC) recommendations. I tell them again that the decision is theirs, but I recommended proceeding with all the immunizations today (a total of five vaccines, but because we use combination vaccines, the baby will only get two shots and one oral vaccine). The parents ultimately decide to proceed with the recommended vaccines, and I provide them with the vaccine information statements for each of the vaccines and tell them to call me with any questions. I feel good that even though the visit took some extra time, I was able to help the parents ultimately reach the best decision for their child.

2:15 p.m.

A 12-year-old boy comes in for his semiannual asthma evaluation. The asthma nurse has already obtained his history and *spirometry* and entered the data into his chart. When I review his chart, I notice that he has been diagnosed with intermittent asthma. However, he has had to refill his rescue inhaler twice last year, and his asthma control test, a standardized asthma assessment tool, shows that his asthma is not under good control. His spirometry also does not look the best. The shape of the curve is fairly convex, and the forced expiratory volume in 1 second to forced vital capacity ratio (FEV_1:FVC) is only 75 percent of predicted, both of which indicate asthma that is not well controlled. I examine him, and he has mild wheezes throughout his chest. I have the patient use two puffs of his albuterol inhaler and have the nurse retest his spirometry. His repeat spirometry looks much better. I discuss this with my patient and his mother. It looks like his asthma should now be classified as persistent, and I explain that he now needs a controller medicine, the most effective of which is an inhaled corticosteroid. I explain how the inhaled steroids are much safer in the long term than repeated oral steroids because the inhaled steroids are deposited mostly in the lungs, and only a very small amount enters the systemic circulation. I give him a sample of an inhaled steroid, as well as an asthma action plan, and schedule him to return to see me in 1 month for a recheck. The rest of the afternoon is fairly uneventful, spent seeing a variety of patients ranging from newborns to college kids with a great variety of complaints.

5:30 p.m.

Prebaby class. Once every week or so, we host a class at each of our offices for expectant parents. We use this as an opportunity to introduce our practice to prospective parents and let them know what to expect after their baby is born. We cover topics such as fever in the newborn, immunizations, *jaundice*, breast-feeding, our office services, and phone advice, and we answer any questions the parents have. We also half-jokingly invite them to stock up on sleep the next few weeks before the baby is born because they will be sleep-deprived after the baby arrives. It is great to experience the expectant sense of wonder, anticipation, and marvel at their impending arrival with these parents. The class lasts for about 30 minutes, and we have several thoughtful questions from our five families tonight. I head home for dinner.

8:00 p.m.

Society for Physician Assistants in Pediatrics (SPAP) conference call. After eating dinner with my family and helping my wife put our girls to sleep, I dial in for my final call of the evening. As AAPA liaison to the AAP, I also serve as a volunteer on the board of directors of SPAP. The call mainly focuses on logistics surrounding our upcoming annual CME conference, which is only a few days away.

Working as a PA in pediatrics is extremely rewarding, challenging, frustrating, and enjoyable, all at the same time. As with any job, some days are harder than others, but most days are really good. For most of my career I have sought opportunities to learn new things, become professionally involved, and give back, and I think that it has served me well. Most important, I always put my patients first, and I remember that is why I work in pediatrics. As the AAP motto says, I am "Dedicated to the health of all children."

A DAY IN THE LIFE: OTORHINOLARYNGOLOGY (ENT)

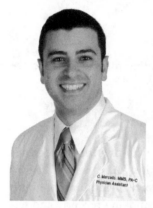

Jose C. Mercado, MMS, PA-C

The adult and pediatric otorhinolaryngology Ears-Nose-Throat (ENT) practice I work for has three offices in culturally and economically diverse locations. We travel between offices daily because it affords us the opportunity to see and treat a broad spectrum of adult and pediatric ENT disorders. The medically underserved patient population in South Florida makes each day unique. One minute I am speaking half Spanish and half Creole to the family of a 2-year-old girl with chronic ear infections; the next I am continuously bowing my head with an 89-year-old Chinese patient while her grandson translates her complaints of nasal obstruction. We typically see patients of almost every ethnicity, ranging in age from newborn to well in their nineties. Symptoms include ear and sinus infections as well as head and neck tumors. Fortunately, we have the ability to perform complete audiometric evaluations as well as fiberoptic endoscopies in the office. This allows us to quickly and efficiently diagnose and treat these common ENT conditions.

6:50 a.m.

My day begins in the intensive care unit (ICU) checking in on a 46-year-old man with respiratory failure who is scheduled for a *tracheostomy* this morning. After reviewing the chart and making sure that labs, consent, and all paperwork are in order, I ask the nurse to call for transportation while I round on the remaining patients. I come back in time to help the nurses transport the patient to the operating room (OR).

7:30 a.m.

While the anesthesiologist and nurse are receiving the patient, I make sure that the OR is ready. After working with my supervising physician for over 10 years, I like to anticipate what he needs before he asks for it. The tracheostomy procedure goes smoothly, and the patient is transferred to the recovery room in stable condition. I then make my way to the office while my supervising physician performs an adenotonsillectomy and bilateral *myringotomy* with ventilation tube insertion on a 9-year-old girl with chronic ear infections and obstructive sleep apnea.

8:30 a.m.

I arrive early at the office to begin tackling the waiting messages and to see the first wave of patients.

9:45 a.m.

My third patient of the day is a 48-year-old man who presents for consultation of a clogged left ear with resulting hearing loss. After a brief history and physical examination, I notice his hoarse voice. I inquire about his alcohol and smoking history. He tells me he quit smoking recently and has been hoarse for several weeks. After removing the wax from his ears and resolving his initial reason for today's visit, I then direct my attention to examining his vocal cords. Topical anesthetic and decongestant are applied intranasally, and a complete *fiberoptic* nasal *endoscopy* reveals a large *pedunculated*, irregular lesion on the left true vocal cord. This is highly suspicious for malignancy. We discuss the risks, benefits, and alternatives to microlaryngoscopy with biopsy. I order the appropriate computed tomographic (CT) scan of neck, chest x-ray, and dental evaluation in preparation for his surgery and subsequent radiation therapy if the biopsy is positive. He is scheduled for a follow-up with my supervising physician once tests are complete and before surgery.

10:30 a.m.

A 19-year-old woman accompanied by her mother presents with complaints of a left neck mass that has been getting larger despite being on oral antibiotics for 3 weeks. On physical exam I note a round, smooth, fluctuant cyst along the left sternocleidomastoid muscle. We discuss the differential diagnosis, which includes a lymphoepethial cyst, brachial cyst, necrotic lymph node, and possible malignancy. Mother and daughter discuss in Creole, and they request to proceed with an in-office fine-needle aspiration. Initial aspiration yields copious cystic fluid. I repeat the procedure with an 18-gauge needle and aspirate 9 cc of fluid, and the cyst is gone. The patient will return in 2 weeks to discuss pathology results and to review results of additional blood work to include a complete blood count (CBC) and human immunodeficiency virus (HIV) test. Both the patient and her mother understand that depending on these results, further diagnostic tests may be necessary as well as surgical intervention.

11:15 a.m.

I drop by the ICU to check on our tracheostomy patient and talk with his family before driving 30 minutes to our other office.

12:45 p.m.

My first patient after lunch is a familiar face. He is 46-year-old man with hypertension, allergic rhinitis, and recurrent nosebleeds. As I pull out his makeshift nasal packing made from toilet paper, he apologizes for not being able to stop his nosebleed. After identifying the site of his anterior *epistaxis*, I cauterize it with *silver nitrate*. We again review instructions for future nosebleeds. He understands that his allergies and sneezing are only part of his problem. He needs to control his hypertension and agrees to follow up with his primary-care physician.

1:20 p.m.

Next up is a 4-year-old girl who returns for follow-up exam for otitis media. She was first seen 2 weeks ago after failing a screening *audiogram*. After I removed her cerumen impaction, I noticed that she had bilateral middle ear *effusions*. We had talked about treatment options, including bilateral *myringotomy* with ventilation tube insertion. The mother elected a final course of oral antibiotics and eustachian tube exercises. Unfortunately, there has been no change to her middle ear effusion, and her audiogram confirms a 35-dB conductive hearing loss. Mom elects to proceed with outpatient surgery for ventilation tubes.

4:50 p.m.

My last patient of the day is a 68-year-old Hispanic woman with a 3-week history of vertigo. She states she went to the emergency room (ER) last weekend, where a CT scan of brain was negative. She was sent home on meclizine, which she discontinued because it made her very sleepy and did nothing for her dizziness. Her symptoms are worse when she turns her head to the right but resolve after a few minutes. On physical exam, there is no middle ear effusion; audiogram confirmed normal age-appropriate hearing. Her neurologic exam is nonfocal. The Dix-Hallpike maneuver is positive for benign paroxysmal positional vertigo. After explaining the reason for her vertigo, I get her set up for physical therapy and canalith repositioning. The patient left in improved spirits.

On an average day, I may see between 25 and 35 patients of almost every age with almost every type of ear, nose, and throat problem. Another joy of practicing in adult and pediatric ENT is that we can usually make everyone better with medicine or with surgery.

José C. Mercado, has been a PA with Dr. Scott Goldberg and South Florida ENT Associates in Miami, FL, since 2001. He is a fellow and past president of the Society of Physician Assistants in Otorhinolaryngology/ Head and Neck Surgery (SPAO-HNS). He serves as adjunct faculty at Miami-Dade College and Barry University's Physician Assistant Programs in Florida. The author has no relationships to disclose relating to this piece.

A DAY IN THE LIFE: ORTHOPEDIC SPINE SURGERY

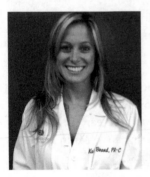

Katherine Ann Boand, MS, PA-C

I am an orthopedic spine surgery PA at Cedar Sinai and St. Johns Hospital, which provides a large variety of experiences both inside the operating room (OR) and in the clinic setting. The change of scenery keeps my job challenging and rewarding.

Education and communication play a large role in my job description during clinic hours. For most patients, the spine is a terrifying subject because of lack of knowledge about spinal anatomy. A large percentage of people in their lifetime suffer from a spinal condition.

As first assistant in the OR, I play an instrumental role in each case and relay pertinent details to patients and their families. My OR time is an exciting and fulfilling part of my job.

6:45 a.m.

I arrive at Cedar Sinai Hospital on a Monday morning. The main lobby is welcoming, warm, and upbeat. Hospital employees surround the coffee shop and are ready to start their day.

I am anxious and excited; hours of preparation have gone into making sure that this day runs smoothly. As I walk into the preoperative area on the eighth floor, my first patient is waving at me. I greet him, and our banter continues because we have developed a rapport over the last year of his treatment.

"How are you this morning? Do you remember what we are doing today? Are you still experiencing primarily leg pain?" His posterior lumbar region is signed in order to clarify the correct site of surgery.

This white-haired old man is one of my favorite patients. He is a 93 years old and suffers from severe spinal stenosis causing symptoms of *neurogenic claudication* and *radiculopathy*. His quality of life has decreased significantly, and he is now unable to sit, stand, or ambulate for a long period. He is ready to undergo an L3–S1 lumbar bilateral *laminotomy* and decompression.

7:20 a.m.

While the OR nurses are performing intake for the upcoming case, I walk down the eighth floor hallway to the inpatient hospital rooms. I converse with the nurses regarding our patients' advancement and then round on our patients from the previous Thursday–Friday OR day.

There is a 34-year-old man who underwent an L4–L5 artificial disk replacement with posterior microdiskecotomy. By postoperative day (POD) 4, he is ready for discharge. He initially presented with severe lumbar pain and right leg pain. He had a *degenerative disk*, an annular tear, and a right-sided herniated nucleus pulposus. His surgery was successful, but his postoperative course was complicated by an *ileus* on POD 2 despite his motivation and efforts to use as little narcotics as possible.

After treatment with Reglan suppositories and a nothing by mouth (NPO) diet, he improved and is now ready for discharge.

Down the hall is a 65-year-old woman on POD 5 from a T3–pelvis posterior spinal fusion, *laminectomy* L1–S1, and L2 *osteotomy*. Her severe *kyphoscoliosis* has been corrected, and her leg pain is much improved. I pull her Hemovac drains out and let her know that she will most likely be going to a rehabilitation center in a few days.

The next postoperative patient is a 58-year-old man who underwent a L2–L4 *laminectomy* and fusion. After everything he has been through, I admire his sense of humor. He jokes with me, saying that he is ready to start gymnastics! I discharged him today on POD 4 and reminded him— *no* bending, twisting, or lifting.

After rounding, I head back to the OR, where the first case is about to start. I review all the patient's history, x-rays, and magnetic resonance imaging views (MRIs) with my attending physician. Once the patient is intubated and lines placed, the positioning of the patient begins.

8:20 a.m.

I'm scrubbing outside the OR with my attending physician. After 4 years of working together, he has groomed me into the surgical PA that he wants me to be. The rapport between PA and attending is important, and the friendship we have developed over time helps us to trust each other professionally. I have been blessed to start this job at a young age and now finally feel confident in my role.

I learn spine care not only from my attending but also from the other PAs with whom I on a day-to-day basis. Bouncing ideas off one another and conversing about difficult cases aids me in my knowledge and interpretation skills.

Many of the OR staff (anesthesiologist, nurses, and scrub technicians) have been there for years. This team working together plays an intricate role in facilitating the start time of each case. Working long hours together brings us closer and makes even Mondays great.

8:30 a.m.

Once we are gowned and gloved, the incision is made. I aid in the exposure of the lumbar spine for the first hour. Once the spine is exposed and levels are confirmed, the microscope is brought in. During the decompression, the surgeon is alleviating the stenosis meticulously, which takes time because we are working on a 93-year-old spine.

During this 4-hour case, although always serious, we are able to discuss our upcoming week of patients and surgeries.

11:30 a.m.

Closure of the wound commences. I take my time with the patient's wound because this is the superficial aspect that will be exposed and shown off to friends.

12:00 Noon

The patient is in the recovery room. After testing his motor strength, I tell him and his family that the surgery went well and without complications.

1:00 p.m.

The next patient is anxiously waiting in the preoperative area. She is a 24-year-old woman undergoing a *microdiskectomy* for her L5–S1 *disk herniation* causing left +4–5 plantar weakness. Her injury occurred in a car accident 6 months prior, and she attempted conservative therapy without success. I bring her family back and again reassure them and discuss the risks and benefits of the procedure. It is not uncommon for patients to show anxiety prior to surgery; it is part of my job to help ease those fears.

1:30 p.m.

This case was quick. The level was identified, and exposure was completed. Under the microscope, the surgeon removed a large piece of disk that had herniated and was compressing the nerve root. The patient was sent home a few hours later with a lumbar corset and pain medication.

3:00 to 7:00 p.m.

Our next case is a 48-year-old woman needing an anterior cervical *diskectomy* and fusion (ACDF) of C4–C7 after experiencing *myelopathic* signs of spinal cord compression. Her balance has been worsening, and she displays upper extremity hyperreflexia. She is unable to lift her arms to brush her hair, has difficulty walking, and is having weakness in her triceps and with wrist extension. Her MRI showed congenital cervical spinal stenosis with level 3 degenerative disk disease and a disk herniation at C6–C7. Her 3-hour surgery is a success.

7:00 p.m.

After a long but rewarding day, I sit back in the recovery room. After answering various phone calls regarding medications, concerns, and pain, my day is almost done.

I reflect on what an amazing field I am in. I enjoy the OR for the technical challenges. Getting to know each patient prior to surgery makes the experience of his or her recovery more personal. Although I am not a surgeon, I believe that my role as a PA has positively affected their lives.

I have the luxury of being able to work while many of patients are suffering from debilitating spinal conditions. I feel lucky to be able to live my life without pain.

A patient gave my attending physician a gift of a simple license plate stating, "I've got your Back."

A DAY IN THE LIFE: UROLOGY

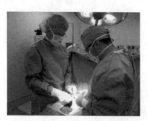

Todd J. Doran, MS, PA-C, DFAAPA

Getting to work is always a challenge at a large university medical center. We are located downtown with large parking lots for employees away from the medical center. I get my exercise walking from the parking lot instead of taking the shuttle. The Oregon air is humid in the summer and windy in the winter. Carrying an umbrella is a sign of weakness if you're an Oregonian; however, it's a sign of a wise southerner. You never know when a flash thunderstorm will dump on you. I traverse up and down stairs and dart between buildings because I've learned all the shortcuts to arrive the back way into clinic. My attending, Dr. Milam, is on vacation this week, so I'm holding down our practice. Our team has been together for 9 years along with our nurse, Peggy Shuster.

8:30 a.m.

My first consult is a 36-year-old man for infertility with severely low sperm counts. The records are being requested while I take his history and examine him. History reveals that he smokes marijuana daily and drinks alcohol on a regular basis. These historical items are newsworthy to his wife, who is present. His exam is remarkable for bilateral soft 15-cc testes, both vasa present, and the absence of a palpable *varicocele*. Records arrive and confirm a semen analysis with normal volume, low counts, and poor motility. We develop a plan to stop drinking and smoking marijuana and a repeat semen analysis after abstaining for 90 days. Serum testosterone, leutenizing hormone (LH), and liver function tests (LFTs) are pending. The patient will notify my office if he has problems quitting which will prompt a referral to a substance-abuse counselor, which he declines today.

10:00 a.m.

The next patient is a 69-year-old man who was last seen 2 years ago with a history of an artificial urinary sphincter (AUS) placed by Dr. Milam. He has been followed locally for a 6-month history of intermittent, symptomatic urinary tract infections (UTIs), and an indwelling Foley catheter was placed recently for increasing urinary incontinence, all history unknown to us. I remove his Foley catheter and deactivate his AUS so that he can be set up for *cystoscopy*, which I have privileges to perform. Cystoscopy confirms my suspicion that the cuff of his AUS has eroded into his urethra. I discuss with the patient and his wife that he needs to have his AUS removed and urethra repaired. This is stage one of a two-stage procedure. His replacement AUS will be delayed at least 3 months until he recovers from the first surgery. This is scheduled for the week Dr. Milam returns from vacation, and a quick call to him confirms the plan.

12:45 p.m.

Clinic has once again run over into the lunch hour due to a host of factors: registry staff, attending on vacation, and add-on procedures. I'm used to this, and it's part of a busy practice. I dash down to the cafeteria and grab a bite. My clinic starts at 1:00, and I have until about 1:15 to eat.

1:15 p.m.

A 56-year-old diabetic man with a history of Peyronie's disease and erectile dysfunction (ED) is referred to our practice, and he has driven 3 hours with his wife to be here. Peyronie's disease is a poorly understood disease with abnormal acquired curvature of the penis with pain and accelerated erectile dysfunction due to scar tissue in the corpus cavernosum. He should have been put into Dr. Milam's clinic but somehow is mistriaged into mine. I examine him, and we discuss the risks, benefits, and alternatives to an inflatable penile prosthesis, and he is booked for surgery. He will meet Dr. Milam when he shows up for his pre-anesthesia appointment that must be completed within 30 days of surgery. A happy patient leaves with a treatment plan. We have run this drill before, reinforcing the principle that Dr. Milam and I are one team.

4:45 p.m.

I've just finished up with my last patient, and the new second-year resident asks me to look at a postvasectomy semen analysis to confirm *azoospermia*.

Now it's time to get caught up on phone calls, lab tests, and dictations. This is my third academic urology job, and I take my academic responsibilities seriously by speaking regularly on areas related to my expertise, as well as being a board member of the Urological Association of Physician Assistants (UAPA). I'm drawn to the patient complexity that is referred to a place with a reputation like Dr. Milam's and Vanderbilt University's. I also enjoy the continual opportunities to learn and teach others. Our team truly improves the quality of life of the patients we see.

A DAY IN THE LIFE: UROLOGY: FEMALE PERSPECTIVE

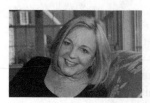

Wanda C. Hancock, MHSA, PA-C

After 12 years in the field of urology, I still have never regretted entering the specialty. Urology typically has been considered a man's world. However, many urology patients are female and would prefer seeing a female physician assistant (PA) or doctor for their care and management. Some urology PAs practice clinically, others practice surgically, and some do both. My practice is in the clinical setting with procedures done as the need arises.

8:15 a.m.

The day begins with chart review of the new laboratory results and imaging reports. Many of the labs reveal rising prostate-specific antigen (PSA) values—those with known prostate cancer will be considered for additional treatment; the others will require a biopsy. I also review cytology reports, computed tomographic (CT) scans, and notes from primary-care providers. There are many decisions to make before I start seeing patients.

8:30 a.m.

My first patient is here for benign prostate hypertrophy (BPH) and lower urinary track symptoms (LUTS). At his last visit, I prescribed an alpha-blocker, and his symptoms have improved. I perform a digital rectal examination (DRE) and order a repeat PSA blood test, and he is scheduled to return in 6 months.

Next, I see a 30-year-old woman for chronic pelvic pain. Her in-office urine sample is clear (without blood or bacteria), and she has no complaints. I refill her medications and schedule her repeat appointment for 1 year.

8:45 a.m.

A 50-year-old woman is referred here for her metabolic workup for chronic *nephrolithiasis*. Imaging reveals no new stones and no enlargement of her lower-pole stones. I review her labs and decide on dietary and medical management of the high calcium level in her urine. In 6 weeks we will reassess the urine and her tolerance of the treatments.

I have a 15-minute break to catch up on chart dictations and phone calls.

9:10 a.m.

My next patient, a 60-year-old man who is here for a Lupron injection for treatment of his prostate cancer. He complains of urinary urgency and frequency. His medications are reviewed and urine is tested. He has an infection and has residual urine present in his bladder after voiding. I perform a DRE. The prostate is likely infected, as shown by tenderness and gland enlargement. The cancer nodules are still palpable. I prescribe an antibiotic. He will return in 4 weeks for a repeat urinalysis and again in 6 months for another injection.

9:25 a.m.

A 30-year-old man comes in for a suprapubic catheter change. He will require lifelong catheter placement because a spinal cord injury (SCI) caused neurogenic bladder. Initially, a Foley catheter was placed, but it was complicated by urethral erosion requiring a suprapubic catheter. During our clinic appointment, I perform *cautery* on the *cystostomy* to remove granulation tissue. We will see him again in 4 weeks for another catheter change.

9:30 a.m.

The next appointment is follow-up on chronic *orchalgia*. The patient has been treated with antibiotics and oral steroids with only minimal improvement in his pain. I explain the risks and benefits of the next-best treatment, the direct injection of steroids into the cord in the testicle. While the nurse prepares the procedure, I have the patient sign the consent form. The procedure goes smoothly, and he will follow up in 4 weeks.

In the next hour, I see three female patients for chronic urinary tract infection (UTI) follow-up.

10:50 a.m.

The paperwork is finally finished for the 10:30 new patient. Ms. Perkins is an 80-year-old woman with a history of urinary incontinence, microscopic hematuria, dysuria, and constipation. She is using several pads during the day and recently has had *enuresis*. On physical exam, she has suprapubic tenderness. Her pelvic exam reveals atrophic vaginitis with erythema, vaginal discharge, *cystocele*, and *rectocele*. A measurement for *postvoid residual* reveals 260 mL of urine. I counsel her to increase her water and decrease her caffeine intake, and I explain Kegel exercises and Crude maneuvers. I prescribe Diflucan, topical estrogen, and stool softeners. She has multiple medical problems, including diabetes and atrial fibrillation;

therefore, surgery is not the best option given her age, her anticoagulation therapy and delayed healing secondary to diabetes. We will follow up with her in 4 weeks to see if her symptoms have improved.

11:45 a.m.

A postoperative patient is added to my schedule because of problems with voiding. She is 4 days postoperative from a midurethral sling procedure by one of our surgeons. Her postvoid residual in the office today is 200 mL. Her incision is healing, and she appears stable. She will return in 1 week.

12:00 Noon

Another patient is added urgently to my schedule, a 40-year-old man with diabetes and a new scrotal abscess. I examine the patient to find a localized abscess without obvious signs of necrosis. My assistants get supplies while I prepare my local anesthetic. I perform the incision and drainage, pack the wound, and write a prescription for antibiotics.

12:30 p.m.

A luncheon begins about the details of a new drug on the market. The presentation is interesting, but it cuts into my free time to dictate my morning charts.

1:15 p.m.

The next patient is a 67-year-old man who recently underwent a coronary artery bypass and is here for a voiding trial. Following his surgery, he was unable to void and comes in for removal of his Foley catheter. His catheter is removed, and his DRE reveals a normal prostate. I instruct him to return if he does not void within 3 hours and return for follow-up in 1 week to measure his residual postvoid.

1:30 p.m.

Mr. Dixon comes in for his regular annual follow-up. We review his laboratory results and assess his medications. He has cancer of the prostate that has been stable since *brachytherapy* 2 years ago. The PSA today is elevated. Examination of the prostate is normal, and the prostate has shrunk since his last examination. He is provided reassurance and scheduled to come in again in 3 months for a recheck. His *nocturia* and urgency have increased, so medications are started to ease his symptoms. He is encouraged to call us if his symptoms do not improve within a week.

2:00 p.m.

A 17-year-old girl comes in as a follow-up from the emergency room. She was seen 2 weeks ago for a ureteral stone that she passed successfully. I am sending her stone for analysis so that we can prevent the development of new stones. She has a low level of discomfort in the left flank area and a trace of blood on urinalysis. We obtain an ultrasound to ensure that her *hydronephrosis* has resolved. She is given reassurance and dietary instructions.

The next three patients are here for follow-up on their medication response to LUTS. Most are managed effectively with alpha-blockers. One of the patients has an abnormal prostate examination, so I refer him for a transurethral ultrasound (TRUS) biopsy.

3:10 p.m.

Another new patient arrives for evaluation of stones. I review her CT scan of the abdomen and pelvis to find a 7-mm *calculus* at the right ureteropelvic junction. After I consult with my supervising physician, I proceed with scheduling the patient for surgery. It is unlikely that she will pass the stone, so analgesics, antiemetics, and an alpha-blocker are prescribed. All the options for management are discussed, and she elects *ureteroscopy*. The history and physical exam (H&P) are completed, and the patient is sent for scheduling.

4:00 p.m.

All the patients are finished for the day. I review the labs and complete my dictations. With all the paperwork finished, I make a few phone calls to report results to patients.

On the way home, I reflect on the day and feel a true sense of comfort knowing that I provided good, ethical, and considerate care to all my patients. Being able to offer patients the tools to feel better and the empowerment to stay healthy is a great part of my role as a PA.

A DAY IN THE LIFE: FAMILY PRACTICE

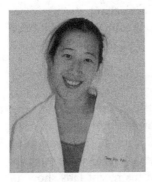

Tammy Woo, MPAS, PA-C

I enter the large three-story medical plaza building. Our office is neatly decorated and is themed for this Fourth of July. The office manager, my medical assistant, and I catch up on our upcoming holiday weekend plans as we log onto our computers. I scan through my phone messages, new labs, and test results. After a few phone calls to patients regarding results, I am ready to start seeing patients.

8:00 a.m.

My first patient of the day is a 64-year-old diabetic man who has recently suffered a mild stroke. His nephrologist manages his blood pressure due to his comorbid renal insufficiency. Today, he complains of right knee pain. On exam, his knee is stable, without evidence of infection or effusion. I order an x-ray, recommend rest, ice, compression, and elevation (RICE), and prescribe pain medication. He is scheduled to follow-up in 1 month, sooner if his knee pain worsens.

9:00 a.m.

Next, I see a 16-year-old girl with a chief complaint of sore throat and fever. She has four out of four Centor criteria: history of fever, absence of cough, tender anterior cervical adenopathy, and white tonsilar exudates. I prescribe penicillin. I advise her to do saltwater gargles and take ibuprofen for her pain. Her mom asks about getting her tonsils out, but for insurance reasons, we cannot refer to ear, nose, and throat (ENT) after a first-time occurrence. After her mom steps out, she quietly asks me if I do Pap smears. I tell her yes, quickly ask her if she needs birth control, and we schedule her for next month.

10:00 a.m.

The next 2 hours are filled with healthy patients with simple chief complaints such as medication refill, urinary tract infection (UTI), and upper respiratory tract infection (URI).

12:00 p.m.

I have a 1-hour lunch break. Occasionally, I have to chart, discuss cases with my supervising physician, or return phone calls. But most days I can go out to lunch or run errands.

1:00 p.m.

I see a 24-year-old man with a chief complaint of chest pain after an intense workout session. After I take his history, perform his physical exam, and see his normal electrocardiogram (ECG), his diagnosis leads more toward musculoskeletal chest pain than cardiac chest pain. He has no chronic medical conditions, no family history of heart disease, and his recent labs show an excellent cholesterol profile. If his symptoms change or continue, I encourage him to go immediately to the emergency department. He is to follow up in 2 weeks or return sooner if his symptoms worsen.

3:00 p.m.

My supervising physician is quite lenient with my patient scheduling. I generally see patients every 15 minutes, but I have the freedom to have longer appointment blocks when I deem necessary. My next patient always gets 30 minutes. She is an 82-year-old woman who treats our monthly visits more as an afternoon tea rather than a medical consult. She annually sees a cardiologist, nephrologist, and gastroenterologist for her chronic hypertension, hyperlipidemia, mild renal insufficiency, and gastroesophageal refluc disease (GERD). I monitor her monthly labs, refill her medications, and reassure her because she is a hypochondriac. Last month it was her toe fungus, the month before it was a tickle in her throat, and the month before that was a fear that her hair was getting thinner. Most of the time she simply needs a bit of reassurance; other times I might order some lab work. Her nail culture results did grow a fungus, and she asks about a remedy she saw "advertised on TV." But I discourage her from trying the medication because of its potential side effects of liver damage and her advanced age. Only one nail is affected, and it is mild. Today, her complaint is dry mouth. Her thyroid test from her labs done 2 months ago is normal. I review her medications and am unable to isolate any particular cause. I then proceed to ask her about over-the-counter medications and alternative medicine use. She states that she has been taking an allergy medication. I tell her that might be the cause of her dry mouth and also advise her to see her dentist to get additional recommendations. She thanks me for my time and promises to bring pictures of her grandchildren next month.

3:30 p.m.

My next block of time is spent seeing patients who called today for a "same-day appointment." I see a 22-year-old with an ankle sprain, a 35-year-old with epigastric pain, a 5-year-old with ear pain, and an 18-year-old with insomnia.

5:00 p.m.

Before I know it, the day is over. I stay an extra 15 minutes because my last patient was running late, but most days I finish on time. I mentally review my day and make sure that I have followed up with all tests and returned all my phone messages.

The best part of my job in family practice is building special bonds with patients and growing with them through the years. I contrast my seasoned 3-year relationship with some patients to my budding relationship with the 16-year-old who shyly asked about Pap smears. It is very satisfying having such a rewarding career that allows me to help people while creating long-term relationships from all facets of life.

A DAY IN THE LIFE: PROCEDURAL PA IN THE EMERGENCY DEPARTMENT

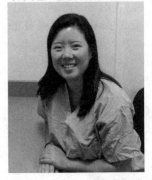

Sarah Esther Hwang, MPAP, PA-C

My first job after graduation from physician assistant (PA) school was in emergency medicine. What I enjoy most is procedures. I am a hands-on type of person, and luckily, laceration repairs and incision and drainage procedures are the bread and butter in the ED. I am now in my second job as a PA and fortunate enough to be in an unusual position where my primary responsibility is to do procedures for the entire ED. If there are no procedures needed, I still see my own patients.

3:00 p.m.

I walk into the locker room and change into my work scrubs. Next, I meet with the PA who is going home. He gives me reports on his patients, who are now my responsibility. On my way to my assigned area of the ED, a physician colleague stops me and asks if I can repair a self-inflicted wrist laceration. I begin to repair the wound. To lessen anxiety, I usually like to explain the procedure and inform the patient of what is occurring while I do the repair. But as I am exploring the wound to assess the depth of the laceration, the patient casually asks me if she had cut herself deep enough. I hesitate and reassure her that it does not look serious. She then asks me if I can point out where her arteries are located. I look at the patient, give a polite smile, and decide quietly that in the best interest of this patient, certain information should not be shared.

4:00 p.m.

Once I am finished with the laceration repair, I sign up for two patients who are waiting to be seen. My scribe, who documents my notes for me, accompanies me as I see my first patient, who is a young woman lying on the gurney curled up in a ball and grimacing in pain. She has right flank pain, fever, and vomiting. Her physical exam, labs, and urinalysis suggest that she has a kidney infection. I order intravenous fluids, antibiotics, and pain medications. I move on to my next patient. She is a middle-aged woman brought in by paramedics for neck pain secondary to a motor vehicle accident (MVA). I clear her from the backboard, leave the cervical collar on, and order cervical x-rays.

The unit secretary informs me that I am needed for a procedure. I find the ED physician requesting my assistance. He tells me that a middle-aged man presented with a headache for the past 5 days. The patient does not have a history of headaches, and the computed tomographic (CT) scan of his head is negative. A *lumbar puncture (LP)* is needed to rule out a *subarachnoid hemorrhage*. I introduce myself to the patient and make sure that he has consented to the procedure. As I gather my equipment, I interview the patient. His headache began suddenly, and because no over-the-counter (OTC) medication improved his pain, his wife insisted he go to the ED. As I insert the needle between his vertebrae, I feel the telltale "give," and I know that the needle is in the right place. When I pull the stylet out, there is a return of pinkish fluid. This indicates blood in the cerebral spinal fluid (CSF). The physician's suspicion is confirmed. When I am done collecting the

CSF, I see a *xanthochromia* layer forming in the tubes, further validating the diagnosis of subarachnoid hemorrhage. I communicate these findings to the physician.

5:30 p.m.

My new patient is a 3-year-old boy brought in for fever who is active and running around the exam room. I imagine this patient returning to the ED in the future for a minor head injury. The patient's mother is concerned because the boy had a runny nose all day and suddenly developed a fever. I examine the hyperactive child and inform his mother that the most likely diagnosis is a viral infection. She seems dissatisfied with the diagnosis and asks for an ibuprofen prescription.

It's time to reassess both patients that I originally saw at 4:00 p.m. The patient with the kidney infection is feeling much better and has passed her PO challenge. I discharge her home with a prescription for antibiotics and pain medications. The patient with neck pain has negative x-rays. She feels better, and I discharge her with a pain medication prescription. I struggle with the feeling that I am giving out pain medication too liberally. In retrospect, each case demonstrates a legitimate need for pain control.

6:30 p.m.

For the next few hours I see patients with minor injuries, abdominal pain, coughs, and chronic pain. It would not be a typical day in the ED if there is not at least one patient with chronic pain asking for a "pain shot" and a prescription for pain medications. I try to stress the importance of having their chronic condition managed by one provider instead of seeing a different provider every time they come into the ED, but many of these patients do not have easy access to their primary-care doctors or do not have health insurance.

9:30 p.m.

After my break, I see a 70-year-old woman with right elbow pain. While celebrating her birthday drinking several mixed drinks of orange juice, vodka, and Bailey's Irish Cream, she tripped and landed on her elbow. Her x-rays show an elbow fracture-dislocation. I'm hesitant to sedate her because she still has alcohol in her system. Instead, I distract her and quickly pop her elbow back into place before she can register what is happening. A splint is applied by an ED patient-care assistant (PCA), and the postreduction x-ray reveals that her elbow is back in place.

My next patient is a 13-year-old boy who injured his knee during a football game. The knee appears disfigured but does not appear dislocated on physical exam. Unfortunately, the x-rays show a distal femur fracture that goes through the growth plate. I ask the unit secretary to page the pediatric orthopedist at the local children's hospital.

The secretary informs me that I am needed to do another LP and laceration repair. One of the more challenging aspects of my job is to prioritize my workload. On one hand, I do not want to make the ED physicians or the patients wait too long for me to do procedures, but on the other hand, I do not want to delay a treatment plan for one of my own patients. I assess what needs to be done first and decide that I need to first finish taking care of my patient with the broken femur. I discuss the case with the pediatric orthopedist, and he asks to have the patient transferred to his facility for surgery. An ED PCA helps me put a splint on the leg, and the patient is safely transferred to the children's hospital.

10:30 p.m.

I find the patient who needs the LP. Unfortunately, the patient is a neonate with a fever. My most successful solution for a quick and nontraumatizing LP is to find an experienced ED PCA who knows how to hold a newborn and to use a pacifier coated in liquid sugar.

Next, I go to the patient needing the laceration repair. While I'm repairing the laceration, another unit secretary asks me if I can return a phone call from one of the hospitalists. There is a patient who is being transferred to the intensive-care unit (ICU) from another floor of the hospital, and he needs a central line. I don't usually venture outside the ED, except to the cafeteria, but once in a while I will get called into the ICU.

Time-consuming procedures, such as putting in a central line, are one of the main reasons why the procedural PA position was created. A procedural PA can allow the ED physicians to maximize their time and see more patients by delegating certain procedures to the PA. For instance, one of my more memorable cases was a patient with a facial laceration from an assault with a broken wine bottle. The repair required more than 30 stitches and took about an hour. It was a delicate procedure that demanded a great deal of dedicated time, care, and patience. Because I am performing procedures frequently, I have become confident and efficient.

12:00 Midnight

I go to the ICU with my supplies and find my patient. Using the ultrasound, I insert the central line catheter into the right internal jugular vein. A chest x-ray is ordered to confirm placement of the catheter.

I return to my desk and thank my scribe for her hard work. Just as I can free up my supervising physician's time, my scribe saves me hours of charting and dictating. At the end of each shift, I review my charts, add a short paragraph if needed to explain my medical decision making, and sign it electronically.

1:00 a.m.

It has been a long day, but I am satisfied with the work I have accomplished. I let all the stress from today's work melt away as I walk to my car. Tomorrow, I have the day off, and I am planning on fully enjoying the warm San Diego sun.

A DAY IN THE LIFE: PSYCHIATRY

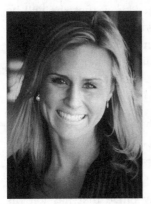

Brynn Bailey-Van Sluis, MS, PA-C

The sun rises brilliantly each morning in southern California. Waves crash on the shore, birds sing, and the world comes alive. Unfortunately, some people do not see these miracles. Their world is often sad, disorganized, and confusing. Each individual is unique and has a life story that shapes his or her current situation, whether it is new or he or she has struggled with it for years. I work as a psychiatric physician assistant (PA) in Laguna Beach, CA. Throughout the day, I visit with people on all paths of life who could be your mother, father, husband, wife, sibling, grandparent, or best friend.

8:00 a.m.

I start the day at the behavioral health unit seeing inpatients for new psychiatric consultations. My first patient is a 24-year-old man admitted last night for depression and a suicide attempt. He is soft-spoken and states, "My family is better off without me." He has been struggling with depression for several years following a traumatic motor vehicle accident that has left him with gross facial deformities. "I'm a monster." He feels hopeless, worthless, and angry. He complains of chronic pain due to his injuries. He recently increased his use of alcohol, consuming to "black out." He has been arguing with his parents, which led him to overdose on Dilaudid and Valium. I place him on a 5150, which means that he may endanger others or himself and requires him to stay for medication management and counseling. I will contact his family for further information.

9:00 a.m.

The next patient I see is a severely disorganized 36-year-old woman who has been diagnosed with schizoaffective disorder. She has bright pink and green hair, neon-orange fingernails, several tattoos, and facial piercings and is half-dressed in a hospital gown. She is angry and yelling at me for being in "this hell hole." She has been off all medications for several weeks and has had increasing paranoia as well as auditory and visual hallucinations. She explains that she has to get out of the hospital to "debug" her apartment. She continues to ask if she is being videotaped during her interview. Her speech is rapid. She has not slept in days. I do my best to calm her down and let her know that she will be staying for further evaluation. She is unhappy with that decision. I leave her room as she demands we discharge her "now!" I restart her on a mood stabilizer and antipsychotic medication and put her on "one-on-one" watch, meaning a staff member in the unit will sit in her room and watch her all day.

10:00 a.m.

I travel up the elevator to the recovery center for additional psychiatric consults. There I first see a 45-year-old man with a history of alcoholism and depression. He has been through an 8-day binge that has left his teeth stained with red wine. He looks exhausted and frail, and he has gross tremors. His eye contact is poor. He has been drinking at least three bottles per day for several years. He complains of chronic pain due to a history of gastrointestinal issues. He has poor social support, financial struggle, and a meager living situation. I will continue his detoxification and start him on an antidepressant.

11:00 a.m.

Next is a 28-year-old woman 11 weeks postpartum. She complains of suicidal thoughts and alcoholism. She drinks a fifth of vodka daily. She feels guilty owing to her irresponsible parenting and appears very hopeless. She recently wrote her husband a suicide note. He brought her to the hospital for evaluation. She has several superficial cuts on her wrists and arms—some are scabbed over and others are fresh. She admits to cutting behavior over the last several months. She is upset with her husband for "forcing" her to come to the hospital. She does not want to be away from her infant. Sobbing, she pleads for help. I reassure her that we will do our best to stabilize her so that she can become a better mother. She is thankful and at ease before I leave.

11:30 a.m.

I head to the staff lounge, where I write and dictate a detailed note on each patient, finish any orders, make necessary phone calls.

1:00 p.m.

I transition to my outpatient office after lunch. A young man I have been following up with for a few years is in the waiting room. I call him into my office. He informs me that he recently started college and feels that he could benefit from attention-deficit hyperreactivity disorder (ADHD) medication again because he has taken a break on it over the summer. He is struggling with procrastination and feels very disorganized. He explains that he is constantly misplacing things and has been late to several of his classes. He has been on a stimulant throughout his school years and has noticed a great improvement while on medication in the past. I restart him on a low dose of a stimulant to use as needed and have him follow up in 1 month.

1:30 p.m.

A very excited and bright 42-year-old woman is pleased to tell me that she is feeling "much better." This is her first follow-up in 6 weeks after starting medication for a long history of anxiety, which has gradually worsened over the years. She had never been treated in the past. "I feel like myself again!" She is able to drive without fear, function in a social setting, and is enjoying life. She has not had any panic attacks since our last visit. Her irritability has decreased. Her family notes a "big difference." In addition, her ongoing history of abdominal discomfort has diminished. She leaves my office with a medication refill and a smile.

2:00 p.m.

A new patient accompanied by her husband fills out her paperwork in the waiting room. I call them back and explain that I will be going through a thorough history today. The patient informs me that she was recently discharged from a psychiatric unit for her first manic episode. She had a sudden onset of poor sleep, which lasted for several days. She was elated, euphoric, hyperverbal, artsy, irritable, and extremely impulsive. She drove to Las Vegas and had a one-night stand. She racked up her credit cards and was drinking alcohol excessively. Her husband brought her to the hospital once she returned home. She is stable at this time and denies any manic symptoms. Her mother died 3 months ago, which has been a great stressor. She denies any mental health issues prior to this year. She was started on lithium in the hospital and now feels "normal." She is afraid that she will have another episode. She feels intense guilt and embarrassment. She is concerned about returning to work in a social setting. I encourage her to stick with the mood stabilizer and start a partial hospitalization program to get some daily therapy for a few weeks. I order labs to check her lithium level. Her husband is supportive and reassures her that he will not leave her. They leave my office holding hands.

3:00 p.m.

An established 23-year-old patient is next. She hasn't followed up with me in approximately 4 months. Last time I saw her, she was stable and enjoying life. She was on a combination of two antidepressants at that time. She was doing so well that she decided to discontinue one of them. She has noticed gradual decline since then, complaining of poor appetite, decreased motivation, low energy, poor focus, decreased libido, hopelessness, and *anhedonia*. She realizes that she was doing better on both medications. I restart her medicine and encourage therapy as soon as possible.

3:30 p.m.

A follow-up with a young military wife is next. She has been on Zoloft for a history of anxiety. She has been stable, although she is apprehensive about the future. Her husband will be deploying soon, and they may have to move. She has three small children and no family or friends nearby. She worries about the "unknown." I encourage her to start counseling therapy and continue her on her current dose of Zoloft. I schedule a follow-up for 3 weeks, after her husband has been deployed.

4:00 p.m.

My last new patient of the day is a 56-year-old woman with a history of panic disorder and *trichotilomania*. She has recently pulled off all of her eyelashes and most of her eyebrows. She complains of psychosocial stressors such as marital problems, unemployment, and financial stress. Her son recently went to jail for drug abuse. She has been depressed and is having panic attacks daily. She is isolated and fearful to go out in public. She is currently on a selective serotonin reuptake inhibitor (SSRI), which has had some benefit in the past. I increase her dose and encourage frequent cognitive-behavioral therapy.

As my day closes, I am thankful for the encounters with my patients. I am driven daily by the opportunity to help others deal with profoundly personal issues by listening, counseling, providing resources, and prescribing medication. I thoroughly evaluate their family history, childhood influences, social environment, medical history, and personality disposition.

I am continually challenged and rewarded with my career as a PA. I pray that I am able to make my patients more comfortable and well adjusted. I hope they function better and see the colors of the world brighter. I will forever be fascinated with the mind.

A DAY IN THE LIFE: BURN CENTER

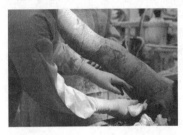

Scott Blow, MPAS, PA-C

When I was a student in physician assistant (PA) school at the University of Florida, I never imagined that I would work in a burn center. This was one of those medical subspecialties that was discussed but never truly covered in depth. By no means am I the first PA to work in this field; I'm just one more in a line of dedicated professionals striving to improve patient care in this challenging medical subspecialty.

I work at an American Burn Association/American College of Surgeons–verified regional burn center in Florida, where I treat all types of burn wounds. Many of our patients are referred to us from other hospitals, emergency departments, and physician offices. I work with a team of clinicians that includes an attending physician, a burn fellow, three plastic surgery residents, and an advanced registered nurse practitioner (ARNP).

5:30 a.m.

I arrive early and round on all of my patients for the day. I check the daily list of patients and see that we had some new admissions overnight. A 23-year-old white man who was burned during an airplane crash is in the burn intensive care unit (ICU). He fell 200 feet, and amazingly, he suffered only a broken clavicle. His burns, however, cover 75 percent of his total body surface area (TBSA) and appear to be mostly full-thickness injuries with some circumferential burns on his extremities. I know that his wounds, fluid status, and pulses will have to be closely monitored for the next several hours to assess for *compartment syndrome*. After his wounds are *debrided*, I apply silver sulfadiazine cream and cover the burns with a dry gauze dressing. A sobering way to start any morning.

6:30 a.m.

I meet with my team for pre-rounds prior to walking rounds with the attending physician. We discuss overnight events and how our patients are doing. The meeting is brief; then we divide up the orders that need to be written, patients who need to be transferred or discharged, and the services we need to consult for our patients before entering the operating room (OR).

7:30 a.m.

Our first OR case is a 34-year-old white man who had attempted to burn some brush with gasoline and a lighter 4 days ago. The fumes ignited and caused a flash-flame burn injury. He has a 10 percent TBSA burn to his bilateral upper extremities and hands that initially appeared to be a mix of partial- and full-thickness injury; through serial wound examinations, we determined that he would need skin grafting. After seeing the patient and checking his labs, we take him back to the burn OR. The patient is sedated with general anesthesia, and after he is prepped, we begin the process of excising the burn wounds. I begin tangential excision on one arm, while the burn fellow works on the other arm. Because these surgeries can be very bloody, we always make sure that we have cross-matched plenty of blood for our patients. We use a mixture of tourniquets, tight-gauze wraps, and a thrombin spray to achieve *hemostasis* on the extremities. While waiting for this to occur, we use the dermatome to harvest skin grafts from the patient's thighs. A *dermatome* can slice an extremely thin layer of skin, about 0.010 to 0.012 inch thick. This patient has plenty of donor sites, so we can use a sheet graft instead of a meshed skin graft. Meshed skin grafts can leave a poor cosmetic result and may provide less wound contraction. After we finish, I help transport the patient to the postanesthesia recovery unit and inform the family that the surgery was a success.

9:45 a.m.

The team is ready to begin our next case, a 42-year-old white woman who was burned on the job. She is employed as an electrician and was burned when the wire she was working on ignited, resulting in a flashback fire. She sustained partial-thickness burns to 12 percent TBSA on her face, right upper extremity, and bilateral lower extremities. She will undergo wound debridement and *xenograft* placement. Xenograft is a biologic dressing, usually made from pig skin, that acts as a scab. It allows the wound to epithelialize, prevents the loss of moisture, and protects against infection; 1 to 2 weeks later, it is removed. Usually, patients with a xenograft have less pain and are able to go home with minimal wound care in a couple days.

11:00 a.m.

Once a week the entire team meets for *interdisciplinary* rounds with representatives from adult and pediatric critical care, infectious diseases, nursing, pharmacy, neuropsychology, physical and occupational therapy, nutrition, social work, and chaplain services. We outline full treatment plans for all our patients at this meeting. Every member of the team provides vital information on how well a patient is healing and what needs to be done prior to discharge. Once the meeting is over, the burn fellow and I take care of what needs to be ordered (e.g., consults, labs, medicine changes, etc.) and which patients need to be scheduled and prepared for surgery this week.

12:15 p.m.

I meet briefly with the research assistant who helps coordinate new and current studies being conducted at the hospital. She informs me that the institutional review board has just approved our next study, which is on the use of *stem cells* to treat partial-thickness thermal burn wounds. The trial will compare spraying stem cells on burn wounds with applying normal saline to burn wounds. There is always something new, and we are excited to be involved in the development of a product that can improve patient care.

1:00 p.m.

I grab some lunch and head to the burn clinic. My first patient is a 3-year-old African-American girl who was getting her hair braided when she accidentally leaned back too far and hot water spilled down her back. *Scald* injuries are the most common type of burn injury in pediatric patients; luckily, this little girl only suffered a 4 percent TBSA partial-thickness injury. It's been 2 weeks since her burn. I remove the dressing to find that her burn wounds have fully epithelialized, and they are only slightly hypopigmented at this time. I instruct her mother to keep the patient out of direct sunlight, give them some moisturizing cream to apply to the healed area, and "medicate" the child with a sucker for being such a good patient today.

2:30 p.m.

After seeing several other patients, my next patient is a 23-year-old Hispanic man who suffered a 23 percent TBSA thermal burn wound approximately 12 months ago. He underwent excision and skin grafting to cover his wounds. He has been doing well at home and has been going to outpatient occupational therapy for a hypertrophic burn scar contracture across his right elbow that significantly limits his range of motion. On examination, I see a hyperpigmented, raised hypertrophied scar and find that his elbow extension is decreased by about 15 degrees. The patient states that he has difficulty at work when using the arm. I make an appointment for him for next week to be evaluated by my attending physician for possible surgery to revise the scar.

3:45 p.m.

My last patient today is a 56-year-old Hispanic man who was referred to the burn clinic for follow-up by another emergency department in the area. He was cooking with grease 2 days ago and suffered superficial burns to his bilateral lower extremities. I evaluate his injury and see that the burn is strictly superficial. I assure him that the wound is similar to a minor sunburn and should be better in about 1 week. He can use moisturizers or aloe vera cream to soothe the affected area.

4:45 p.m.

While finishing my clinic, I receive an urgent page to return to the burn ICU. The nurse informs me that the patient with the 75 percent TBSA burn has lost the pulses in his right lower extremity despite adequate fluid resuscitation. I alert the fellow and attending, who meet me at the bedside immediately. We attempt, unsuccessfully, to Doppler any pulses in the extremity. The leg is pale in appearance, and the nurse says she had to increase the patient's sedation to keep him comfortable. We decide that the best course of action is an emergent *escharotomy* of the leg to relieve the pressure that has accumulated secondary to the injury and swelling. The fellow and I use an *electrocautery* device to release the compartments of the leg along the lateral aspect of the extremity. We can see the leg opening up as the pressure is released with each cut of the device. On reassessment of the distal pulses, we find that they have returned and are adequate.

6:00 p.m.

This has been another long, eventful day, and I am ready to go home. I make my final rounds and write my postoperative assessments. I am told that sometime during the night the unit will receive a 31-year-old African-American woman from an outside hospital with suspected Stevens-Johnson syndrome after taking an antibiotic. According to the outside facility, she has approximately 45 percent TBSA open at this time. I know we will need to be ready for almost anything when she arrives. After finishing my remaining dictations, I head off to dinner with my girlfriend and some friends.

Scott Blow works at the Tampa General Hospital Regional Burn Center, Tampa, FL. He has indicated no relationships to disclose relating to the content of this piece.

Reprinted, with permission, from the *Journal of the American Academy of Physician Assistants*, December 2009.

A DAY IN THE LIFE: NEONATAL INTENSIVE CARE UNIT

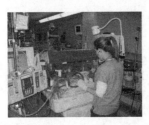

Shana Perman, PA-C

Once I learned about the physician assistant (PA) profession, I knew it was the profession for me. After graduating from the PA program at the Philadelphia College of Osteopathic Medicine in 2005, I started my first, and current, job in the neonatal intensive-care unit (NICU) at the Children's Hospital of Philadelphia (CHOP). I knew that I wanted to work in pediatrics. My only previous NICU experience came during my elective rotation in PA school, but CHOP was willing to hire and train new graduates. I work with a front-line clinician group consisting of PAs, nurse practitioners (NPs), and house physicians. My work schedule includes days, nights, and weekends—every day is different, yet exciting.

7:00 a.m.

I arrive at CHOP and get sign-out on my patients (there are seven today) from the overnight front-line clinician. One of my patients, Baby M, a 4-month-old former 26-week preemie, had increased abdominal girth, irritability, and a low-grade fever overnight. She is postoperative day 2 after G-tube placement and Nissen *fundoplication* for severe reflux. We see a lot of former preemies who need these procedures because of severe gastroesophageal reflux that can cause worsening lung disease. I record the overnight and morning lab results on all my patients. I also learn that I will be getting a new admission from an outside hospital today.

7:30 a.m.

I examine my patients and review their flowsheets for the past 24 hours. A lot of numbers are involved in the patients' day-to-day care: new weight for the day, how many grams up or down from the day prior, total fluid intake, urine output per hour, respiratory support, blood pressure (BP), abdominal girth, scores to assess pain, and any apnea, bradycardia, or oxygen desaturation events.

Baby M has already had a blood and urine culture done overnight and is started on vancomycin and gentamicin for a *septic* rule-out. I give her a dose of fentanyl for pain and update the surgical team that performed her procedure.

8:30 a.m.

My front-line group meets to look at the radiographs from the morning and start bedside rounds—a total of 17 babies today. We go over the previous days' totals with the attending and decide on our plan for the day. After consultation with the surgical team, the decision is made to send Baby M for an upper gastrointestinal (GI) study through her G-tube to make sure that the tube is in the correct position and there is no leak. She is scheduled for 2:00 p.m. Because Baby M is no longer intubated from the surgery, her nurse will take her to the study; patients who are intubated must be accompanied by a front-line clinician.

10:00 a.m.

I receive a page informing me that my new admission has arrived, so I leave rounds to go to her bedside. The transport team signs out that the ambulance trip was uneventful and gives me a copy of the records from the outside hospital. My new patient is a 2-day-old infant girl who was born via C-section at 37 weeks because of worsening bilateral *hydrone-phrosis* that was diagnosed on ultrasonography at 24 weeks' gestation. I examine the baby and enter admission orders. After consulting with the urology and nephrology teams, I order a renal ultrasound and a voiding *cystourethrogram*.

10:45 a.m.

I rejoin my team to finish rounding. Another one of my patients is Baby S—a full-term boy who had significant respiratory distress at birth and was intubated for 5 days. He has since been extubated and is working on feeding by mouth. Babies with feeding difficulties are seen by a speech therapist, who is at the bedside to talk about Baby S's progress. The therapist would like to schedule him for a modified *barium swallow* in the next couple of days to assess his feeding ability and to make sure that he can be fed safely by mouth.

11:00 a.m.

The ophthalmology team notifies me that one of my patients, Baby C, is going to need laser eye surgery this afternoon. Baby C was transferred to CHOP because of worsening *retinopathy* of prematurity. The condition is thought to be caused by disorganized growth of retinal blood vessels and, in serious cases, can result in blindness due to *retinal detachment*. Baby C is currently only on a nasal cannula for respiratory support but now needs to be intubated for the surgery. Her parents are at the bedside, and after ophthalmology gets consent for the surgery, I talk to Baby C's parents about intubating her.

11:30 a.m.

I update the attending about Baby C's eye surgery and then enter orders in the computer for the rest of my patients.

12:15 p.m.

While eating lunch in my work area, I type the admission summary for my new patient. Luckily, she's only 2 days old, so her records from the outside hospital are minimal. Since most of our patients are transferred from other hospitals, we often get 3- or 4-month-old former preemies with multiple medical problems and a stack of paperwork that you cannot imagine! While most of our patients are born at other facilities, CHOP recently opened a special delivery unit where mothers can deliver babies with known birth defects; these babies are a small percentage of our patients. Currently, there are approximately 65 beds in the CHOP NICU, but we are making renovations to accommodate more patients.

1:00 p.m.

One of the nurses pages me that another one of my patients, a 10-day-old 24-week preemie, has worsening blood gas results compared with her previous numbers. This baby was transferred to CHOP a couple of days ago for an intestinal *perforation* after receiving indomethacin to treat her *patent ductus arteriosus (PDA)*. The PDA needs to be treated if it is causing an overcirculation of blood to the lungs. I go to the patient's bedside, increase her ventilator settings, and order a STAT chest radiography. The radiograph shows that her endotracheal tube is a little high, so it is adjusted and retaped. A follow-up blood gas with the adjusted endotracheal tube and increased ventilator settings shows improvement.

2:00 p.m.

Baby M's nurse lets me know that my patient is back from her upper GI study. Thankfully, Baby M's G-tube is in the correct position, and there is no leak. The surgical team is notified. Baby M will stay on antibiotics for a 48-hour septic rule-out.

2:30 p.m.

I order the rapid-sequence medications that will be given to Baby C prior to intubating her for eye surgery. We try to intubate a baby a couple of hours before surgery to allow time to make any necessary adjustments to the endotracheal tube and ventilator settings. When the nurse and respiratory therapist are ready, I go to Baby C's bedside to intubate her. There are no complications; a chest radiograph will be done to confirm placement of the endotracheal tube. Baby C is placed on the ventilator and will have a blood gas drawn to make sure she is stable on the current settings. Her surgery will start early this evening at her bedside. The front-line clinician on call for our team will be there during the surgery and will sedate Baby C. The surgery can take 1 to 2 hours when both eyes need to be done, as is the case for this baby.

3:15 p.m.

When I call to let Baby C's nurse know that the endotracheal tube is in good position, she reads me the blood gas results. They are good—no ventilator adjustments are necessary. I update the summaries for two of my patients who will likely be discharged home in the next couple of days.

4:00 p.m.

The overnight front-line clinician comes in, and I give her sign-out on each of my patients, including any labs for tonight and the following morning.

4:30 p.m.

Baby S's nurse pages me. The patient's parents have arrived and would like an update. I talk to the parents about the barium swallow requested by the speech therapist. I will call them tomorrow when I know the scheduled time for the study.

5:00 p.m.

I leave the hospital and turn off my pager. Days like these seem to go by quickly and can be draining at times. As with any other area of medicine, there is a constant learning curve. Even though the NICU can take an emotional toll on all involved, the best reward is seeing a baby get better and go home.

Shana Perman works in the Division of Neonatology at the Children's Hospital of Philadelphia and the Hospital of the University of Pennsylvania in Philadelphia. She has indicated no relationships to disclose relating to the content of this piece.

Reprinted, with permission, from the *Journal of the American Academy of Physician Assistants*, August 2009.

A DAY IN THE LIFE: CARDIAC CRITICAL CARE

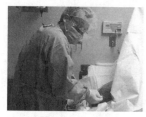

Robert G. Baeten II, MCMS, PA-C

About 3 years ago, I began a unique position as a cardiac critical-care physician assistant (PA) at the esteemed Piedmont Hospital, a rapidly growing tertiary-care facility in Atlanta, GA. My PA teammates and I practice at the hospital with a high degree of autonomy, especially after hours. On a daily basis, we manage critically ill patients, perform procedures at the bedside, and provide a central-line service for the entire hospital. Besides caring for cardiology patients in the intensive-care units (ICUs), the other PAs and I also help to manage patients in the cardiothoracic, vascular, and thoracic surgery departments.

6:55 p.m.

I arrive at the hospital to begin the critical-care night shift. My day-shift counterparts give me sign-out on our ICU patients, and my phone starts ringing before the shift begins. Already I can tell it will be a busy night. We are short-staffed, so I will be working alone tonight. The nurse on the phone describes a problem with a coronary-care-unit (CCU) patient and requests a prn medication. Midway through our conversation, call waiting interrupts, and I switch over. It's the emergency department (ED) reminding me to admit a patient for chest pain. After finishing sign-out and wrapping up the CCU nurse's request, I admit the chest pain patient. Luckily, this admission is straightforward, and I submit orders and finish dictating the history and physical examination before the next call comes in.

7:40 p.m.

The phone rings three times in a row. I have a patient to see in the CCU, a cardiology consult for *bradycardia* in the oncology unit, and a central line to put in for a patient in the ED. I go first to the patient who needs the central line. I discuss the procedure with him and assess the ideal position for placing the line. This particular patient is *septic*, has stage IV chronic kidney disease, and is on warfarin for atrial fibrillation (AF) with an international normalized ratio (INR) of 3. I decide to go in through the left internal jugular vein with direct ultrasound guidance. The line goes in smoothly, and I order a chest x-ray to confirm proper placement. While awaiting the images, I get a call that the patient awaiting a cardiology consult in the oncology unit has heart block.

8:20 p.m.

I run up to the oncology unit and review the telemetry strips. The patient has progressed from Mobitz type II to intermittent complete heart block. His labs are normal, and he is not receiving any negative *chronotropes*, but he is borderline hypotensive with a mean arterial pressure of 60 mmHg. I notify my attending cardiologist and the admitting oncologist that I will be transferring the patient to the cardiac intermediate unit and that a temporary pacemaker may be needed tonight. After intravenous (IV) isoproterenol (Isuprel) fails, I have a nurse bring pacing supplies. Meanwhile, I confirm placement of the central line in my previous patient's x-ray and then immediately begin to place a temporary transvenous pacemaker in my current patient. I choose a right internal jugular vein approach to preserve the subclavians for a possible permanent device. Once the bipolar pacing probe is in the right ventricle, I determine the capture thresholds and program the external pulse generator. I update my attending physician, write a progress note, and dictate the consult.

9:45 p.m.

The oncology patient is paced at 60 beats per minute and is resting comfortably. I follow up on the CCU patient with rapid AF and then head back to the ED for another chest pain admission.

12:15 a.m.

During a quick break, I hear a call for code blue in telemetry and arrive at the same time as the rapid-response team. We find a nurse already performing chest compressions on a patient who is not breathing. The respiratory therapist "bags" the patient, while another prepares for intubation. I ask the nurse to hold compressions briefly while I check for a pulse. The patient, a 60-year-old man with an *ejection fraction* of 20 percent admitted 2 days ago with a mild heart failure exacerbation, is pulseless, and his rhythm shows ventricular fibrillation. I order the first shock to be given. After a prolonged resuscitation with several shocks and administration of multiple advanced cardiac life-support medications, the patient finally has a perfusing rhythm. We transfer him to the ICU. He remains unresponsive, and after a brief phone call to update my attending, I proceed with the induced hypothermia protocol. In hopes of a good neurologic recovery, I place a cooling catheter via the femoral vein. Then, I place an arterial line in the femoral artery for close blood pressure monitoring. It is clear that this patient is now in florid heart failure and needs careful hemodynamic monitoring. I insert a Swan-Ganz catheter via a right subclavian approach. His cardiac index measures 1.5 and wedge pressure is 30. I order diuretics and an inotrope while discussing ventilator settings with the respiratory therapist before finishing my progress note.

3:00 a.m.

I check on a postoperative day 1 quadruple coronary artery bypass and aortic valve replacement patient who has required increasing pressor support over the last few hours. His hemoglobin level has dropped from 10 to 7 g/dL. I order several units of packed red blood cells (RBCs) and a STAT chest x-ray. Almost the entire left lung field is opacified on the films. The chest tubes placed intraoperatively have not been draining a significant amount. The patient is still intubated but is arousable and appears agitated. Suddenly, a large amount of blood gushes from the chest tubes. I call the cardiothoracic surgeon in immediately. The surgeon takes the patient back to the operating room (OR).

3:45 a.m.

I get a call about a patient in the ED with new-onset rapid atrial fibrillation and a transfer from a rural hospital who will need to be admitted for acute coronary syndrome. I evaluate the patient in the ED and find that his rhythm is actually atrial flutter. His x-ray reveals he has a dual-chamber implantable cardioverter-defibrillator. I retrieve the appropriate device programmer, interrogate the device, and see that he was in sinus rhythm only 8 hours ago. I adjust the device settings to painlessly pace the patient out of flutter back into sinus. The tachycardia has exacerbated his heart failure, so I admit him for diuresis and start heparin. I put in a consult for our electrophysiology service to see him in the morning for possible flutter *ablation*.

4:30 a.m.

The ED notifies me they need a stat Vas-Cath catheter to be placed on a hyperkalemic patient. He has altered mental status and is obese with a body mass index of 51. He has a potassium level of 7.7 mEq/L and a creatinine level of 5 mg/dL, requiring emergent dialysis. Unfortunately, he has coagulopathy with an INR of 4 and a platelet count of 85/mL. Fresh-frozen plasma is infused. The patient's groin has significant skin breakdown, making it a poor choice for line placement. Under direct ultrasound guidance, I place a 14F Vas-Cath catheter in the patient's right internal jugular vein without difficulty. A portable chest x-ray is done, and I confirm proper line placement. *Hemodialysis* is started immediately.

5:00 a.m.

I get more coffee and walk back through the units. My induced hypothermia patient is at the goal temperature and is producing urine. His cardiac index is up to 2.2 L/min/m², and his wedge is down to 20 mmHg. He appears to be improving from a hemodynamic standpoint. Fortunately, the other patients in his unit had an uneventful evening, and some may be able to go to the floor. It's almost 7 a.m., and I'm looking forward to ending this shift.

5:45 a.m.

I spoke too soon. The transfer patient has arrived on a telemetry floor; while at a smaller hospital, he ruled in for a non-ST-elevated myocardial infarction with only a small troponin bump. His electrocardiogram (ECG) shows acute ST-segment elevations in the anterior leads. I call the interventional cardiologist, and 15 minutes later, the catheterization laboratory team has arrived. I escort the patient to the catheterization laboratory and then dictate the history and physical examination.

6:30 a.m.

I watch the procedure in the catheterization laboratory and see that the patient has a 100 percent proximal left anterior descending lesion. My attending revascularizes the vessel by performing a percutaneous coronary intervention, and the patient's chest pain is relieved. My night finally ends as the day shift arrives.

7:40 a.m.

I head home feeling blessed I could help so many people, praying I can rest before my next shift tonight. Fortunately, a second person will be joining me this time.

Robert Baeten is a critical-care PA at Piedmont Hospital in Atlanta, GA. The author has indicated no relationships to disclose relating to the content of this piece.

Reprinted, with permission, from the *Journal of the American Academy of Physician Assistants*, April 2011.

A DAY IN THE LIFE: HOSPITALIST PA

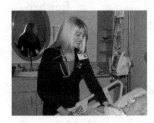

Kristen K. Will, MHPE, PA-C

Like many new physician assistants (PAs), I wasn't sure which specialty I wanted to practice in after graduation. I worked in everything from family medicine to cardiovascular surgery. It wasn't until almost 5 years after graduating, when I accepted a position with a new hospitalist group, that I realized that being a hospitalist PA encompassed everything I enjoyed—high-acuity patients, a team approach to medicine, and a fast-paced environment. Over the past 5 years, I've learned that hospitalist PAs must be able to multitask and prioritize patient care based on acuity while working effectively within the hospital institution as a "system." I admit patients and round on them during hospitalization, write orders, establish care plans, discharge patients, and perform inpatient medical consults for medical and surgical subspecialties.

7:00 a.m.

I arrive at work and page my attending physician, who is carrying the main triage pager for the hospital. During the day, I usually work with four physicians and another PA. This morning, my attending physician assigns me six patients to see. A few I know from the day before, but two were admitted overnight. As usual, their admitting diagnoses are diverse.

I look up all their lab results and vital signs on the computer before starting rounds to see if I need to address any immediate problems. I find that one of my patients became confused overnight with decreased urine output and decide to start with her. This patient was admitted yesterday with an altered level of consciousness from a urinary tract infection (UTI) and has a history of *dementia*. Clinically, she appears dehydrated, so I order a small intravenous (IV) fluid bolus with maintenance fluids along with tomorrow's morning labs. After determining that her antibiotic is still appropriate, I meet with her family. They are concerned that her confusion will not improve, and we discuss acute *delirium* and the prognosis. We also discuss possible short-term placement in a skilled nursing facility after this admission. After our discussion, I make a note to check her urine output and mental status later. I also call social work to come and speak with the family for discharge planning. Continuing through the rest of my morning patients, I examine each patient, write progress notes, order labs, and consult other services as needed. When I'm finished, I check back with my supervising physician to go over the patients I've seen. My attending will visit those patients later, reviewing my note and cosigning my orders.

11:00 a.m.

My attending physician calls me with a consult requested by orthopedic surgery. The patient is an 86-year-old woman with good functional status who fell early this morning in her assisted-living apartment and sustained a left intertrochanteric hip fracture. The hospitalist service has been asked to perform a preoperative medical risk assessment before the patient undergoes open-reduction and internal fixation of the fracture. I quickly review her medical history, laboratory studies, chest film, and electrocardiogram (ECG) on the electronic medical record (EMR), and then I go to see the patient. After taking more history from the patient and family, I perform a physical examination, which is unremarkable except for a grade 3/6 systolic murmur and, of course, the fracture. I recommend to the patient and the surgery team an echocardiogram to rule out significant valvular disease. After completing my dictation and orders, I call my attending physician, who then meets me to review the case and briefly examine the patient. She agrees with my management, and she tells me that after a quick lunch, I should see another new patient—a direct admission from the medical oncology outpatient clinic.

12:30 p.m.

Before I even grab lunch, I call the nurse on the floor to ensure that the new admission is stable and that no immediate orders are needed. After quickly eating, I head upstairs. My patient is a 29-year-old woman currently receiving chemotherapy for invasive cervical cancer, and she has acute onset of fever. Because she is *neutropenic,* she is admitted for a workup and empirical antibiotics. While I am reviewing the history on the EMR, the nurse comes to tell me that the patient is becoming more tachycardic with new hypotension. I immediately go in to see her. She is awake and calm, but her blood pressure (BP) has dropped from 124/74 to 84/58 mmHg. I give a verbal order for the nurse to give a 500-mL IV fluid bolus and to start another IV site. I am worried that the patient is becoming *septic,* and I order STAT blood and urine cultures as well as empirical IV antibiotics. While I'm with the patient, she becomes *lethargic* and more hypotensive. I have the nursing staff start IV fluid boluses wide open in both peripheral lines and in her central line (already in place for her chemotherapy) and call my attending physician. She meets me in the room, and we call for a step-down ICU bed. Unfortunately, the patient is too tachycardic at this juncture to start vasopressors, and her BP remains low. During transfer downstairs, the patient becomes unresponsive. My attending physician and I stay with her while the boluses continue. Finally, after minutes that seem like an eternity, her BP improves, and she becomes more alert, asking, "Oh, hi Kristen—did I go to sleep?" "Yes," I respond, "and you're going to be just fine." I finish writing the admission orders, and then I go to speak with the family.

As a hospitalist PA, one of my main functions is to educate and communicate with patients and families. This is by far one of the most important jobs I do, and it helps to free up my supervising physician to see other patients. This particular case is a good example. Just as I am going to meet with the young woman's family, my attending physician is called about another patient becoming increasingly more ill. She quickly excuses herself to go attend to that patient. After spending over 30 minutes with the family explaining what has happened and the prognosis, I go back to check on the patient. She is awake with a stable blood pressure for now.

1:45 p.m.

I take a short break to follow up on the patients from the morning. My delirious patient is improving, with less confusion and better urine output. I review the echocardiogram on the patient going to surgery and find that her murmur was only aortic sclerosis without stenosis. I call the orthopedic surgery service to say that she may proceed to surgery. After answering some work e-mails, I head back to the step-down ICU to check on my septic patient. Her urine Gram's stain is positive with gram-negative bacteria. Her BP and mentation continue to be stable.

2:30 p.m.

I spend the rest of my afternoon admitting three patients from the emergency department. The first patient is admitted for observation of chest pain. He has no history of coronary disease, but he has many risk factors. His initial cardiac enzymes are negative with a normal ECG. The second patient is admitted for a lower gastrointestinal (GI) bleed but is hemodynamically stable. Before writing her admission orders, I call gastroenterology for a consult; then I complete my orders and dictation. The third patient is admitted for a workup of *syncope*. After each patient, I call my attending physician to review the case and my management plan. My attending then will see each patient later and cosign my orders.

5:30 p.m.

Today, I have a meeting arranged with the chair of the Department of Education for the Mayo Clinic College of Medicine and all the other postgraduate program directors for physician assistants at Mayo Clinic Arizona. I am co-program director of a new postgraduate PA fellowship in hospital internal medicine. We meet to discuss issues that affect all our programs and to go over expectations for the coming academic year. I am excited about our new fellowship! It will be a tremendous experience for the PA fellow and a value to our institution.

6:15 p.m.

Our service is caught up on admissions for now, so I return to check on my patients. The patient with septic shock is doing better, with improved urine output and a stable BP. I review the earlier lab results and make sure that my antibiotic is still the right choice. After speaking with the family and saying good night to the patient, I quickly make my way through the remainder of the patients I have seen today, checking updated vital signs and laboratory findings. I revisit the patient who underwent hip surgery, seeing her in the postanesthesia-care unit. She did well through surgery and looks stable. Lastly, I sign out my patients to the night PA, asking him especially to check on the patient in the step-down ICU. I check with my attending physician one last time, learning that there is no more work for me tonight. I turn off my pager and head for home.

On my way home, I reflect on all my patients today, especially the young woman who became critically ill. I realize that I've made a difference in her life—the very reason I became a PA. Truthfully, it is patients like her who have made a difference in my life. I am thankful that I have found a specialty within my profession that allows me to use my strengths every day to help patients when they need it most. Being a hospitalist PA is challenging and satisfying—and I am excited to go to work each day!

Kristen Will is a hospitalist PA at the Mayo Clinic Hospital, Phoenix, AZ.

Reprinted, with permission, from the *Journal of the American Academy of Physician Assistants*, August 2007.

A DAY IN THE LIFE: HEMATOLOGY

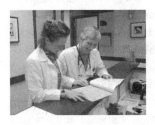

Renee Wittenmyer, PA-C

By Laura Howard, MPAS, PA-C

The Indiana *Hemophilia* and *Thrombosis* Center (IHTC) was started 10 years ago by two hematologists who dreamed of a comprehensive clinic that could meet the needs of patients with benign hematologic conditions. They began hiring physician assistants (PAs) in the spring of 2004 to help them manage the complex medical care their patients required. IHTC is staffed by seven physicians, two nurse practitioners (NPs), and five PAs who manage patients with disorders such as hemophilia, *von Willebrand disease*, thrombophilias, and *sickle-cell disease*. PAs and NPs at IHTC have unique roles requiring expertise in their subset of patients. I follow adult patients with hemophilia who have acquired HIV infection, hepatitis B, or hepatitis C from tainted blood products.

7:30 a.m.

I like to get to work at least an hour before my first patient comes to clinic, which allows me to get caught up on universal data collection reports. These reports are an ongoing collection of individualized patient medical data allowing for documentation for ongoing research and to ensure continued funding for IHTC from government grants and the Centers for Disease Control and Prevention (CDC). My pager goes off as I am entering data. It's a call from a 19-year-old Amish man with severe factor VIII deficiency. A deficiency in clotting factor VIII can cause severe bleeding in soft tissues, muscles, and joints with significant consequences such as *compartment syndrome*, *arthropathies*, or joint deformities.

Hemophilia is an X-linked inherited deficiency of either factor VIII (hemophilia A) or factor IX (hemophilia B). Acquired hemophilia can occur but is very rare. To treat bleeding in patients with hemophilia is theoretically simple: Give them the factor they are deficient in to bring their levels back to normal. Until the early 1990s, replacement factor came from the plasma of people without the disease. The blood was cleaned, but the cleaning process was less than perfect and allowed for the transmission of unwanted viruses, including HIV, hepatitis B, and hepatitis C. At IHTC, we follow more than 300 patients with hemophilia who have acquired one of the aforementioned viruses from blood products received before 1993. Fortunately, *plasma* is now treated with viral-inactivation processes, and recombinant factor is available, both of which have significantly reduced the risk of virally transmitted diseases.

IHTC manages the care of approximately 150 Amish patients with bleeding disorders. Because of their beliefs, the Amish do not carry medical insurance, and the cost of factor replacement can add up to millions of dollars over a patient's lifetime. Many are in a disease management program that provides free treatment; this government program has been shown to save the state millions of dollars when patients are treated promptly after an acute bleed.

8:00 a.m.

I am in an early morning educational meeting when I get paged about one of our patients. He is a 21-year-old Amish man who was kicked by his horse in his left shoulder this morning at 5:00 a.m. He lives 3 hours away and will require factor replacement at 100 percent concentration to minimize the risk of soft-tissue bleeding into his shoulder joint. He is able to catch a ride in a car with a non-Amish friend to a local emergency department (ED) to have his shoulder x-rayed and scanned if needed. I call the ED before he arrives, giving instructions to the charge nurse about how to mix factor replacement before infusion. The Amish man will need to continue infusing himself with factor VIII replacement at 100 percent correction for the next 5 to 7 days. Patients with hemophilia learn how to self-infuse at a young age. Luckily, IHTC's outreach program is going to the town where this patient lives next week, so we will be able to assess his shoulder in person.

9:30 a.m.

Back in my office, I try to catch up on dictations and reports. I am able to get a couple of dictations done before my pager goes off again. I gulp some coffee and dash down the hall to clinic. The patient is a young man with acute intermittent *porphyria*, along with a seizure disorder. He comes in today for a routine exam. Late last year he had a rather complicated hospital course after an acute porphyric attack with subsequent respiratory failure and a *catatonic* state. As I am examining him, he suffers a *grand mal seizure*. I run out of the room to alert the physician and have the clinic nurse call 911. He is brought over to the hospital and admitted for supraventricular tachycardia.

10:30 a.m.

After calling our hospitalist to give him a heads-up on the man with the seizure and ventricular tachycardia, I am paged by Craig, our data coordinator, who reminds me that I have a 10:30 meeting with him and our medical director to review forms and specific links being created for the new electronic medical record (EMR) system. By the time I get out of the meeting, I only have a few minutes to eat a quick lunch.

12:00 Noon

The front-office manager is waiting for me in my office when I return from lunch and asks if I can see a walk-in with a knife wound. The man is 45 years old with severe factor VIII deficiency and transfusion-acquired HIV infection. To date, he has had an undetectable viral load and a CD4 cell count of 600/μL. He has HIV-associated renal failure requiring *hemodialysis* 3 days a week.

When he comes in, I quickly assess the knife wound, which he says he got while defending himself from an attack. He was stabbed on the left posterior aspect of his forearm just below the elbow. I learn that he went to a local ED and received factor VIII replacement and wound care including cleaning and stitches. This man is currently homeless and moves from motel to motel. Two weeks before the assault, he was given a tetanus booster in our clinic during a routine exam. During today's visit, he is given more factor replacement and is scheduled to come in for the next 5 consecutive days for more factor replacement to correct his levels to at least 80 percent to prevent further bleeding and allow for adequate wound healing.

1:00 p.m.

My next patient is an 85-year-old man who is coming in to go over the results of his labs and abdominal computed tomographic (CT) scan. He was at the clinic last week for evaluation of a chronically elevated white blood cell (WBC) count. He recently moved to a nursing home because he has Alzheimer's disease, and he has a history of alcohol dependence. The man's son and daughter-in-law come with him to the appointment today. I discuss the laboratory test results, which show anemia and a low platelet count. The CT scan of his abdomen reveals lesions suspicious for carcinoma. I explain that his liver is probably the site of the primary cancer, with likely metastasis, and provide a referral to an oncologist.

1:30 p.m.

I run back to my office to dictate more notes and get a few more reports done before seeing my next patient. This one is a 42-year-old man here for a routine follow-up visit for anemia from *myelofibrosis*. Today he presents with lower extremity edema and a rash located on his abdomen and groin. The rash appears as a small cluster of *papules* without drainage. This appears to be a side effect of increasing doses of thalidomide. The patient receives a topical cream for the rash and furosemide for the edema.

2:00 p.m.

I meet with a 65-year-old woman who had come in 6 weeks ago for evaluation of an enlarged spleen with borderline low-normal platelet count. CT scan showed an enlarged spleen with displacement of the left kidney. A follow-up cervical lymph node biopsy revealed B-cell lymphoma. I discuss her prognosis and treatment options, and I refer her to an oncologist.

2:30 p.m.

As I am waiting in clinic to review a patient's case with my supervising physician, the triage nurse comes up to tell me that a hepatologist from Indiana University Medical Center wants to talk to me about a patient I sent over for a liver biopsy. After I get off the phone, I go into another clinic exam room to see another patient. He is a 30-year-old man with severe factor VIII–deficient hemophilia with a high responding inhibitor requiring a bypassing agent. Patients with hemophilia can develop inhibitors that block the activity of the recombinant factor VIII product. This makes treating such patients more difficult and more expensive in that they require much more recombinant factor to "overwhelm" the inhibitor. The patient is on the schedule but has shown up 3 hours early with nausea, vomiting, diarrhea, and stomach pain. After a history and physical exam, a severe GI bleed is diagnosed, and the patient is admitted to the ICU.

4:30 p.m.

At this point, I try to keep an eye on the time and wrap up my day. I return phone calls and call patients with lab results, respond to e-mails, double-check the EMR "desktop" for any messages, and dictate the day's office notes. Working at IHTC offers me a rewarding experience as a PA, allowing me to provide multifaceted care to patients with varying *hemoglobinopathies* in the acute and chronic setting.

Renee Wittenmyer practices at the Indiana Hemophilia and Thrombosis Center in Indianapolis, IN. She has indicated no relationships to disclose relating to the content of this piece. The piece was written by Laura Howard, MPAS, PA-C, who is Ms. Wittenmyer's colleague.

A DAY IN THE LIFE: DERMATOLOGY

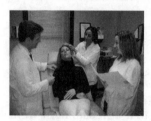

Stephen Steiner, PA-C

I take care of skin for a living. Working in a dermatology practice for the past 7 years, I've grown to appreciate the prevalence of skin cancer, the intractability of an itch that can't be scratched enough, and the heartbreak of an acne flare just before a prom. On any given day, I can see a range of patients from a child as young as a few days old to a frail, elderly woman older than 90 years. Skin is something we all have in common, and unlike many medical issues that are internal, skin is on display for all to see and comment on. While the bulk of my practice involves the medical and surgical management of skin issues, I strive to treat the patient as a whole—mind, body, and spirit.

8:10 a.m.

The morning starts off with a bang. My first patient is an 89-year-old nursing home resident who has been itching for the past 6 weeks. Her son and primary caregiver relate that she has been itching since she started wearing her roommate's clothing. When I ask about the roommate, they remark, "Now that you mention it, she's been itching as well." The skin scraping confirms my suspicion of *scabies*, and I know that I'm going to be itchy for the rest of the day.

9:30 a.m.

After a few mundane cases, I now see a patient who has been dealing with *psoriasis* for the past decade. He is absolutely ecstatic today. About a month ago my supervising physician started him on a new biologic therapy. What numerous creams and pills could not accomplish in years, this new medicine has accomplished in just 4 weeks. His body is nearly free of psoriasis, and he is wearing clothing that he would never have considered before because of the embarrassment he felt over his skin condition. Within the dermatology world, the treatment of psoriasis has undergone a revolution within the past few years. It's an exciting time to be a provider.

9:50 a.m.

One of the nurses knocks on the door and asks me to take a call. She knows that I hate to be interrupted when I'm with a patient, so I know this call is important. She hands me a chart and tells me the dermatopathologist is on line 7. When I submit a biopsy for review, I send along a brief differential diagnosis to assist the pathologist. Every once in a while the dermatopathologist requires a complete clinical scenario to ferret out the diagnosis.

I pick up the phone, and after talking about our golf game briefly, he asks for the background on a patient. I explain that this woman has had a nodular eruption on her shins and a yellowish papule on her forehead. After discussion, we decide her picture best fits *sarcoid*. I'll need to call her this afternoon to set up a chest x-ray and labs.

10:30 a.m.

My next encounter is with an 18-year-old whom I've followed for acne for the past 5 years. She has run the spectrum of acne treatment from topicals to oral antibiotics. She is finally well controlled on birth control pills; they are relatively benign, from my point of view, and she has had no untoward side effects. Her need for me is coming to a close. Instead of focusing on acne during this visit, we talk about her future plans after high school. She is going to college, and I do my best to steer her in the direction of my alma mater. I leave the room with a smile. My role as a friend and mentor has superseded my job as a skin-care provider today. In the grand scheme of things, the conversation we just had far outweighs my boring lecture on the pathogenesis of acne.

11:20 a.m.

I'm about to see my last patient before lunch. I look at the chart before entering the room, and my enthusiasm immediately drops.

This is a 4-year-old boy with warts. I try to smile as I walk in and greet the mother and son. I am met with an immediate outburst of tears and wailing. My worst fears are now realized—and I am about to cry myself. After much cajoling and frustration, I'm finally able to examine the boy closely enough to see that he has six periungual warts. I explain to the mother that warts are viral in origin and have a variable response to treatment. The mother nods understandingly and then states, "Just make sure that they're gone after one treatment. I have a $30 copay, and I don't want to come back just to pay you more money." With these words, an already tough situation gets a bit more difficult. I explain to the mother again that warts have a variable response to treatment, and I simply can't guarantee that the warts will be gone after one treatment. I try to reassure her that I'm not here for profit, and I redirect my attention to the warts at hand.

My preferred treatment for warts is liquid nitrogen. Unfortunately, it's exquisitely painful on the nail folds, and there's a snowball's chance of this patient holding still long enough for me to get an adequate destruction. Not only will I hurt this little boy, but his warts won't go away, and the mother's suspicion of my motives will be confirmed—at least in her eyes. My recommendation is to use a topical *keratolytic* to irritate and debulk the warts, along with a healthy dose of tincture of time. Surprisingly, the mother amenable to this plan, and we agree that I will see her son in 3 months. Hopefully, I can outlast these warts.

12:00 Noon

I have an hour to enjoy my peanut butter and jelly sandwich. I go over the labs and phone calls while I chew. I try to return all patient calls personally, but I simply can't handle the voluminous number of automatically gener-ated refill requests that are faxed from the local pharmacies. I usually leave it up to the nurses to parse out the needed refills from the superfluous.

After all the patient-care issues are taken care of, I stop by the office of one of my supervising physicians. He's just gotten back from a continu-ing medical education (CME) meeting, and I always like to hear about the highlights of the meeting. He does a good job of culling out the critical elements for me; I like to think that I do the same for him.

"I always try to gauge the patient before starting any therapy—I want to maximize the chance of success."

1:30 p.m.

I enter the exam room to find a girl about 12 years old and her well-accoutered mother. Her mother greets me and says that her daughter is here to have a mole on her face removed. I look at the patient and see that she has a 3-mm tan-brown papule on the right malar cheek; there is no evidence of abnormality. There is no medical necessity for this procedure, and as I begin to explain the ABCs of moles, the mother states how much her daughter is mentally traumatized by the presence of this mole on her face. Even the best plastic surgeon would leave a scar that would be noticeable on this cosmetically sensitive area. The daughter has been quiet throughout this whole visit, so I direct my questions specifically to her. Her response couldn't be more surprising. She tells me that the lesion doesn't bother her at all, and it's her mother who wants it removed.

Now I don't have a clue as to whom to believe. Maybe the mother is insisting on this to make her already pretty daughter more beautiful, at least in the mother's eyes; maybe the daughter is deflecting attention and really wants it removed. I suggest that they talk at home about what they really want and what is best for the daughter over the long run. I give them the names of local plastic surgeons and leave the room thinking of Cindy Crawford.

3:30 p.m.

From about this time until the end of the day, my schedule mostly consists of adolescents with acne. I always try to gauge a patient before starting any therapy—I want to increase my chances of success with compliance. I have no doubt that the teenage princess with one small *comedone* will follow my regimen unfailingly. It's the sullen, sulking teen with a combination of papules, pustules, and nodules that I worry about.

I have a love/hate relationship with my teenage patients. Acne is not something that clears quickly, and teens are notorious for demanding immediate results and not following directions (just like adults, now that I think about it). I try to convince them that a clear complexion is the pot of gold that they will be rewarded with time. It's an amazing thing to see that sulking teen who wouldn't make eye contact with me 6 weeks ago turn into an outgoing person with clear skin. Those who blow off zits as a cosmetic condition have no idea about the impact acne can really have on a teenager's self-esteem and social life.

4:30 p.m.

The day is coming to a close. I finish up my dictation and return a few patient phone calls. It has been a good day so far. I worked hard, saw patients with a variety of skin problems, and made a positive impact on their lives. I race out the door and soon find myself at home, where I can devote the rest of my day to the true purpose and joy of my life—being with my family.

Stephen Steiner practices dermatology at Gwinnett Dermatology in Snellville, GA. He has indicated no relationships to disclose relating to the content of this piece.

Reprinted, with permission, from the *Journal of the American Academy of Physician Assistants,* April 2008.

A DAY IN THE LIFE: INTERVENTIONAL RADIOLOGY

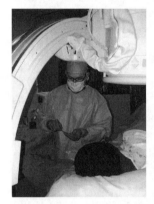

Nicholas Oravetz, PA-C

As a physician assistant (PA) student, I aspired to a high-intensity career in emergency medicine or surgery. I thought that working in one of these areas would let me use all my knowledge and expend all the energy and enthusiasm I had accumulated over 2 years in PA school. Once I graduated, though, I learned that new PAs with no experience have trouble landing jobs of this type. Fortunately, I also learned about interventional radiology (IR) around the same time. I discovered what PAs working in IR at my hospital were doing and how they were used. As a new PA, I had never considered IR and didn't even know that PAs practiced in this field. Luckily, I was offered an excellent opportunity in IR, and to this day, I can't imagine working in a different field of medicine

8:30 a.m.

I arrive at the hospital and am greeted by the usual chaos of patients, staff, and visitors all racing to their destinations. Once in radiology, I meet with the five other PAs I work with to go over our daily assignments. Most of my work involves doing procedures, so I make my rounds through special procedures, *fluoroscopy*, ultrasound, and computed tomography (CT). Because our schedule contains a mix of outpatients and inpatients, we coordinate our inpatients around our outpatient schedule. I visit my first patient in our holding area, an elderly man who needs vascular access in order to begin *dialysis*. Before the procedure, I review the chart, recent labs, medical history, and orders. I talk with the patient about the procedure, and I obtain informed consent. Before starting my first procedure, I check on a few inpatients from the previous day, and I write any necessary orders and a quick progress note for each. This particular day I have only two patients to follow up on, so I finish with enough time to make a trip to the medical staff lounge to grab a quick bite for breakfast.

9:15 a.m.

I'm back in radiology, and the dialysis patient is prepped and draped. After conscious sedation is administered, I begin the procedure. I typically use the right internal jugular vein for a dialysis catheter, given the anatomy and access to the superior vena cava and right atrium, where the tip of the catheter will be placed. The procedure itself takes about 30 minutes, and the patient is transferred immediately to the dialysis unit in good condition.

I move to another room to place a peripherally inserted central catheter (PICC) line, which is a very common procedure for us in IR. I would be lying if I didn't say that placing PICC lines can become mundane, considering the volume of them I do, but the steps are fundamental to almost all the other procedures we do in IR.

9:45 a.m.

By now, the day is in full gear, and an outpatient has just arrived for a CT-guided biopsy of periaortic *lymphadenopathy* found on a prior CT scan. The radiology nurse draws the blood for the necessary lab work (prothrombin time, partial thromboplastin time, and international normalization ratio). Once the results are back, I discuss the case with the radiologist, and we talk over options for the biopsy. The patient is placed on the scanner, and I perform the biopsy, taking special care not to disrupt any vascular or visceral structures, especially the aorta and inferior vena cava. The biopsy sample is obtained, and the specimen is sent to pathology. I write orders for the patient, who recovers in our holding area before going home.

I find it amazing that we can perform such intricate biopsies with such accuracy, but current technology allows us to perform many biopsies that used to require a risky surgical procedure as a relatively safe outpatient procedure.

10:45 a.m.

As I walk back to the office from the CT department, I find myself thinking about the biopsy patient, wondering what the results of the biopsy will be and how they will affect him and his family. I think my work for this reason is meaningful and important. Whether the results are good or bad, patients get some answers about their ailment and can begin the healing process, whichever road that may be. This feeling is common in IR—after all, we PAs are responsible for performing the majority of all biopsies that are done in our radiology department. I am reminded daily of how different patients are from one another and how uniquely their own problems are, but they all have the same human desire to persevere. Beep, beep, beep . . . I hear the all too familiar sound of my pager going off, and my thoughts take another direction. I have two more PICC line patients waiting for me.

11:30 a.m.

We finish early with our morning patients, and I and the other PAs meet back in our office for lunch. During lunch, a patient who had a lumbar puncture a few days ago calls to say that he is having severe headaches. I reassure him, saying that he is probably suffering from a lumbar puncture–induced headache. I tell him that these are an occasional side effect from having this procedure. I phone the anesthesia department and schedule him for a blood patch, which will alleviate his headaches.

The lunch hour gives me and the other PAs a chance to catch up on any developing cases for the afternoon and discuss any interesting patients from the morning. We also go over our inpatient list and review any patients who need lab work before they come down for procedures this afternoon.

1:00 p.m.

The afternoon schedule begins to fill up quickly. A nephrologist tells us about an inpatient who has an occluded arteriovenous dialysis graft. He asks if we can perform a *thrombectomy* to clear the occlusion so that the patient can receive dialysis. I inform the technologists and nurses, and we begin the workup before the patient's arrival. I check the records in our computer system and see that we have done similar procedures on this patient in the past. This information will help us to manage this patient's problems today. The patient arrives, we obtain informed consent, and we prep the patient for the procedure. Using fluoroscopic guidance, I gain access into the graft; using different catheters, guidewires, and a special thrombectomy device, we are able to remove the occlusion. Before the patient leaves the table, I go over my images with the radiologist, and we discuss the case and the outcome. Once we agree that everything looks good, the patient is discharged from our department.

2:30 p.m.

I make my way to the fluoroscopy department and to an outpatient there for a lumbar puncture. I first review prior head studies (MRIs, CT scans) to make sure that the patient has no anatomic variants such as masses that could result in adverse outcomes. Once again, after obtaining informed consent and using fluoroscopic guidance, I perform the lumbar puncture. This patient has a history of weakness and changes in her vision. Her MRI suggested a *demyelinating* process such as multiple sclerosis. During procedures, I often visit with patients, attempting to ease their anxiety and distract them from what's going on. X-ray guidance has dramatically decreased the time and overall difficulty of a lumbar puncture, but I think pretty much everyone, myself included, still appreciates a few comforting words during this type of procedure.

3:20 p.m.

I hurry back to the special procedures department to handle a couple more PICC lines. After this, I have a few minutes to catch up on dictating the procedures performed earlier in the day and to get a little midday fuel in the form of black coffee. I'm sure many readers can relate to the importance of that!

I have just a bit of paperwork to finish and a few more PICC lines to complete on patients admitted from the emergency department. To prepare for tomorrow, I go over the schedule; I present the cases to the radiologist, and we review the appropriate previous radiologic studies.

4:30 p.m.

The workday is complete, and I finish a few last-minute details before heading out the door at 5:00 p.m. This is just one day in IR, and every day is different. Some are hectic and chaotic, but others are quieter. I never know until I get to work what kind of day it will be.

I am fortunate to have found a niche in IR—especially one that allows me a great deal of autonomy but also gives me excellent supervising radiologists who are always willing to help. My experience in IR has proven to be challenging, rewarding, and ever-changing. The need for PAs in radiology appears to be growing; as medicine changes and PAs are introduced into more subspecialty practices, this trend will continue. For now, I head out of the parking garage with only one thing on my mind—enjoying a beautiful Carolina summer evening before I go back tomorrow and do it all over again.

Nick Oravetz works in interventional radiology for Mecklenburg Radiology Associates in Charlotte, NC.

Reprinted, with permission, from the *Journal of the American Academy of Physician Assistants*, October 2007.

A DAY IN THE LIFE: OBSTETRICS AND UROGYNECOLOGY

Barbara Kimmons, PA-C

I would never have guessed that when I graduated from physician assistant (PA) school I would find myself practicing obstetrics and urogynecology. I enjoyed my rotation in ob/gyn, but my focus at the time was cardiology and cardiovascular surgery. When it came time to look for work, though, I could find no local openings in cardiology, so when an ob/gyn position was offered, I accepted the challenge. I practiced as a PA in ob/gyn for 6 years, and I loved it. It is a happy specialty—and definitely not boring or routine, as I thought it might be. My schedule varied depending on surgeries, clinic appointments, and other practice-related obligations, but a typical day went like this.

6:30 a.m.

I arrive at the hospital for a scheduled cesarean section (C-section) early enough to visit with the patient, answer lingering questions, and reassure her about the procedure. Our patient has had a C-section before, but this time she is expecting twins. The ultrasound shows two healthy females. Twin A is in *vertex position*, and Twin B is in *frank breech position.* They are not identical, so each has her own placenta and amniotic sac. The patient's husband is there with his video camera, and Grandma is beaming, as anxious as everyone else to see her two new granddaughters. After talking with the patient and her family, I fill out our preprinted postoperative orders and the operative note before the surgeon arrives.

7:00 a.m.

I meet our patient in the operating room (OR), where I assist in positioning her during the administration of the spinal. Providing comfort and reassurance at this time is a part of my job that I particularly enjoy. I love being first assistant at C-sections because the occasion—bringing new life into the world—is so joyous. Our patient is draped and comfortable with her husband at her side, and the surgeon moves swiftly with the incision, while my job is to retract and suction. Soon the amniotic sac appears, and we see a small head of dark hair inside as we prepare to deliver Twin A. A flood of amniotic fluid helps us to extract the infant; I barely have to push on the mother's abdomen before the baby slips into the world. I clamp and cut the umbilical cord while the surgeon suctions the mouth and nostrils, holds her up for the mother to see, and then passes her off to the neonatal nurse. Now for Twin B. First, the surgeon feels for the position of the baby. Once this is ensured, the sac is broken, and the tiny feet of Twin B appear. Grasping these feet proves to be a challenge—Twin B seems to be crawling back inside where she has been safe and warm for the past 38 weeks. But in an instant the surgeon uses a towel to dry the feet and get a good grasp. Maneuvering the baby's shoulders and head, the surgeon soon delivers her and holds her up for her mother to see before sending her to join her sister with the neonatal team. Cord blood is obtained, placentas are delivered, and the uterus is lifted from the abdominal cavity to have its interior wiped clean before we suture it closed. Once *hemostasis* is achieved, the uterus is returned to its home, and the various abdominal layers are closed. The skin is neatly sutured, Steri-Strips are applied, and we are finished.

8:00 a.m.

While the surgeon completes the notes, I help to clean up the patient and move her to recovery. Next, I'm off to round on other postpartum and postoperative patients. I see all postpartum patients, whether they have had vaginal deliveries or C-sections. These visits are a time for congratulations to the family and gushing over the new baby, but I also check the patient's physical recovery, breast-feeding plans, and *hemoglobin/hematocrit (H/H)* to be sure of hemodynamic stability. I write progress notes and discharge orders, and then I go to another floor to see our gynecology patients, where I check incisions, review labs, check vitals, and write care plans. If there are any consults from other services, I see these patients and dictate histories and physical exam findings for the chart, as well as initiating any diagnostics that may be required.

8:30 a.m.

I arrive in my clinic office, where I review labs, sign charts, and answer urgent phone calls. Today, I have to calm a distraught older patient who had an abnormal Pap test result. We discuss human papillomavirus, and I answer her questions and reassure her as gently as possible. It's almost 9:00 a.m. when I meet with my medical assistant to go over the day's patient list.

9:00 a.m. to Noon

Depending on the day, I may be seeing prenatal and postpartum patients or doing procedures such as *colposcopy*, endometrial biopsy, or *cryotherapy*. I spend most clinic days treating various gynecologic complaints and performing annual well-woman exams. I have the luxury of meeting my new patients in my office, where we can discuss their health concerns in a more relaxed atmosphere than in the exam room. Establishing rapport is crucial in women's health because I may be the only person these patients can come to for support and guidance. I see nervous young couples on the threshold of starting a family, quiet young girls with their anxious mothers, and women of all ages concerned with a myriad of issues. After we have talked, we move to the exam room.

Noon to 1:30 p.m.

This time is supposed to be my lunch break, but more often than not another surgery is on the schedule. Once a month, our office manager holds a lunchtime meeting for all the providers in our practice. We discuss new ideas, patient satisfaction, and, of course, the bottom line. I am also the director of our biofeedback program for urinary incontinence, so at least once a month I use this time to meet with my medical assistant and our biofeedback technician to discuss the program and review the progress of patients currently enrolled in therapy.

Biofeedback is a patented, Food and Drug Administration (FDA)–approved noninvasive program for rehabilitating and strengthening weakened pelvic floor and urethral muscles, thus helping to restore continence, healthy living, and an active lifestyle. Biofeedback translates the contraction from the pelvic floor muscles into a signal that can be seen on a computer monitor. It teaches women how to control these muscles. The program has been very successful for women of all ages suffering from urinary incontinence resulting from a variety of causes, including pregnancy, childbirth, obesity, smoking, estrogen deficiency, and pelvic organ prolapse. We have enjoyed an 85 percent success rate in treating incontinence with our biofeedback program.

1:30 to 5:00 p.m.

The afternoon offers more opportunities for patient education. The topics are varied and include smoking cessation, preventing sexually transmitted diseases, hormone-replacement therapy, oral contraceptive use, osteoporosis, and urinary incontinence. Besides offering the biofeedback program, our clinic performs urodynamic studies. My job is to evaluate the results of these studies and make recommendations before final surgical plans are made. Recently, we have begun screening for interstitial cystitis and performing potassium sensitivity testing for selected patients. In women with interstitial cystitis, the bladder lining is no longer watertight; it has become porous and permeable to the potassium and acids in the urine, setting up an inflammatory process in the muscle of the bladder. Interstitial cystitis can cause chronic pelvic pain, urinary frequency, pain with intercourse, low-back and leg pain, and bladder pressure. Subsequent treatment and monitoring of patients with this condition are another gratifying part of my job. I feel a tremendous sense of accomplishment when a patient's condition responds to therapy, and she lets me know how this has improved her life.

5:00 to 5:30 p.m.

When the last patient leaves, I check my planner for the next day, look at the call schedule to see if I'm on call, clean off my desk, and head home, only a short drive away. My days are full and very gratifying. I am so glad I became a PA, and I'm even happier that I found a niche in women's health. I make a difference in someone's life every day, and at the end of the day, that is what satisfies my soul.

Barbara Kimmons worked in the ob/gyn department at the Sadler Clinic, Conroe, TX, when she wrote this piece. She has indicated no relationships to disclose relating to its content.

Reprinted, with permission, from the *Journal of the American Academy of Physician Assistants*, August 2005.

A DAY IN THE LIFE: TRANSPLANT SURGERY

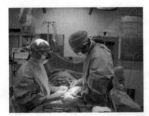

Jared R. Pennington, PA-C, MHS

I began my career as a physician assistant (PA) in 2004, and my first job was in emergency medicine. I stayed for about 6 months until I realized that I wanted to pursue a career in surgery. I'm also a paramedic, and I enjoy taking care of prehospital patients—but I had to move on. My current position in the transplantation department at Geisinger Medical Center has given me a wonderful opportunity to flourish as a PA working in surgery. I have roles as a clinician, a patient advocate, and a researcher, and the combination is what makes my days ever-changing and always exciting. Transplantation is one of those specialties within medicine and surgery where you can actually turn patients' lives around. Freeing patients from *hemodialysis* is one of the greatest rewards.

6:00 a.m.

I start the day by rounding on the inpatients. Today we have five patients on our service, and only one of them is postoperative from last week. Our inpatient list is usually filled with posttransplant patients with urinary tract infections (UTIs) or dehydration. Posttransplant patients who have even the slightest increase in serum creatinine level without a definite cause are admitted to the hospital under our service. We also admit transplant patients who had kidney, pancreas, liver, or multivisceral transplantations elsewhere.

Our postoperative patient in house today underwent a living-related-donor (LRD) renal transplant 4 days ago and is now ready to go home. We frequently transplant kidneys donated by family, friends, or even acquaintances of the patient. Today's patient has membranoproliferative glomerulonephritis (MPGN). This form of *glomerulonephritis* is characterized by thickening and reduplication of the glomerular basement membrane. Type I disease is relatively *benign*, but type II disease is not, and affected patients have an IgG autoantibody. Our patient has type II disease. Patients with type II MPGN usually develop end-stage renal disease (ESRD) over 5 to 10 years.

Our renal transplant patients, particularly the LRD transplant recipients, will spend 4 to 5 days postoperatively in the hospital if all goes well. Patients who receive a cadaveric kidney, however, may have delayed graft function for 5 to 7 days and may need extra time in the hospital with close observation.

7:00 a.m.

Once a week the transplant and nephrology departments have a meeting to discuss annual evaluations of old patients, evaluations of new patients, new transplants, and patients who were recently admitted to the hospital. Many issues are brought to the table during this hour regarding eligibility for transplantation and donor selection.

8:00 a.m.

This is when I go to my office and review the morning laboratory results. Most of the time all the basic labs are back, except for tacrolimus or cyclosporine levels, which usually come in around noon. Tacrolimus is the drug of choice in our program, and it has been shown to be 10 times more potent than cyclosporine. Tacrolimus can cause severe nephrotoxicity with a mild increase in the trough level, however, so monitoring levels is important.

After reviewing the labs, I change intravenous (IV) fluid rates and concentrations, add or discontinue medications, and order laboratory or diagnostic studies for the following day. I also check laboratory data on patients with renal transplants who are scheduled to undergo renal biopsies for that particular day. Most biopsies are done to rule out acute rejection, but some are performed as protocol biopsies throughout the postoperative course depending on the study projects that we're working on.

9:00 a.m.

Rounds begin with the attending surgeon and nephrologist. In transplantation, as in other medical and surgical subspecialties, it is very important to approach the patient as a team. Along with the surgeon and nephrologist, rounds are attended by the transplant nurse, the nephrology pharmacist, the general surgery resident assigned to our service, and me. During rounds, we discuss the patient's progress through the past 24 hours, current medications, risk of infection, and hydration status. In most transplant programs, an hour or more each day is set aside solely to review medication regimens. Posttransplant patients not only take *immunosuppressive medications* but also take *prophylactic* antibiotics to prevent the infections that *immunocompromised* patients commonly acquire.

10:00 a.m.

This is the time when we go into the operating room (OR), if we haven't been there already. One of the surgeons I work with has a great interest in dialysis access surgery, including arteriovenous (AV) fistula placement, AV grafts, and peritoneal dialysis catheter placement. He is the only surgeon in the hospital who performs upper extremity AV fistulas, so we operate on a fair number of patients with ESRD. We also commonly perform permanent hemodialysis catheter placement and Mediport insertions for other services in the health system. Patients are frequently referred to our department from outside and by internal nephrologists for dialysis access. One benefit to having our center perform access surgery for ESRD is that patients have a chance to meet our team before they are placed on our kidney-recipient list when they are in need of a transplant. Most of the time I first-assist on all cases if I am not taking care of a patient inhouse.

We also schedule LRD renal transplant cases throughout the month and typically perform two to four of these per month. I first-assist on transplant cases, including LRD and cadaveric kidney/pancreas transplants. In addition, we perform surgery for portal hypertension, including peritoneovenous shunts, and liver tumor surgery. In March of this year we began a liver transplant program.

1:00 p.m.

After surgery, we review all biopsy results with our transplant pathologist and discuss the results. In almost all cases the patients who underwent biopsy are already being treated if rejection has been found on frozen section or permanent specimen. We bring the biopsy specimens to our renal pathology meeting, which happens once a month, for further review and discussion.

2:00 p.m.

Now the surgeon and I round on our patients for a third time. This is when we adjust tacrolimus or cyclosporine levels based on the results of morning lab tests and check the general progress of the patient. We again assess hydration status and make changes as needed. It is very important to have trough levels of tacrolimus or cyclosporine drawn in the morning because even a small deviation can be detrimental to the patient and/or the grafted organ. We also follow up on any consults that occurred that day.

3:00 p.m.

I return to my office and review journal articles to present to our transplant journal club. I also double-check diagnostic studies and make note of biopsies, surgeries, and clinic patients scheduled for the next morning.

5:00 p.m.

I check my e-mail and talk with the transplant coordinators to see if we are accepting any potential donors in our organ-procurement organization.

5:30 p.m.

Hopefully, by this time, I am traveling a good hour to get home to see my wife, Nicole, our 8-year-old and 9-month-old daughters, Taylor and Olivia, and our dog, Denny. I wish I could say that I won't be returning to work until the morning. Often, though, we will be called to harvest an organ within our six-county region some time during the night. These donated organs may be for one of our own patients or for a patient at another center within our organ-procurement organization.

Transplantation is a busy and demanding field. Overall, however, it is extremely rewarding, with an enormous amount of information to be learned and many patients who need to be provided with the best care possible.

Jared Pennington is the chief PA in the Department of Transplantation and Liver Surgery at Geisinger Medical Center, Danville, PA. He has indicated no relationships to disclose relating to the content of this piece.

Reprinted, with permission, from the *Journal of the American Academy of Physician Assistants,* June 2006.

A DAY IN THE LIFE: EMERGENCY MEDICINE

Jessica Rodriguez Ohanesian, MS, PA-C

On a crisp, cool morning, I walk past employees' vehicles, police cars, and ambulances to reach the doors of the emergency department (ED). Inside is not the typical office setting with paintings on the walls, sweet scents, and coffee handouts. Instead, a middle-aged intoxicated man who smells of vomit, urine, and body odor yells profanities as I pass by. The department is filled with patients in hallway beds and chairs anxiously waiting to be seen. In front of me is the typical shift-switch scene: Half the clerks, technicians, nurses, physician assistants (PAs), and physicians have just arrived looking alert and fresh, whereas the other half look disheveled after 12 hours of hard work. I find my PA colleague, who waits to discuss the unfinished night-shift duties with me—otherwise known as the *sign-out.*

7:00 a.m.

My colleague reports, "A surgical consult is pending on a 45-year-old intravenous drug abuser with arm abscesses likely requiring drainage in the operating room. A 15-year-old girl with bilateral peritonsillar abscesses also has a consult pending. I was unable to complete her incision and drainage and am waiting for a page back from ear, nose, and throat. My last patient is on a psychiatric hold in the behavioral-care unit for a suicide attempt."

My day has now begun. The on-call ear, nose, and throat (ENT) physician arrives to perform the incision and drainage, and I admit the patient for intravenous (IV) antibiotics. The behavioral-care unit calls to have paperwork signed for my suicidal patient's transfer to a psychiatric facility, and the surgical patient is taken to the operating room (OR).

8:00 a.m.

My first two patients are both seeking care for diabetic complications. I start with the 21-year-old woman who received a diagnosis of type 2 diabetes 1 year earlier. She has her arms crossed and phone in hand, scowling, "How long is this going to take?" Her diabetes is poorly controlled with a blood glucose level consistently greater than 500 mg/dL. She proudly states, "I don't care about controlling these levels. I just want to leave. This is taking forever." This particular hyperglycemic episode caused nausea and weakness, and the patient came in to "feel better."

The young woman's hospital neighbor is my other patient, a 47-year-old man with diabetes who fell and is experiencing "stump pain." He smiles as he eavesdrops on my conversation. This patient initially received a diagnosis of diabetes after he presented with bilateral leg paresthesias, which later required an amputation of his left leg below the knee. He is 14 days postoperative and is now here with complications. He lost his balance and fell forward in his wheelchair, causing his stump to bleed relentlessly. Because of his family's concern, he agreed to come in for evaluation. This man's maturity regarding his health issues comes across through his calm demeanor; this is just one of the many ED visits he will likely have for his diabetes issues.

I convince the young woman patient with diabetes to sit with her hospital neighbor while I address his injury. The man speaks words of encouragement to her throughout his wound repair. He tells her, "You want to be able to enjoy your future family, and complications like mine interfere with that and with holding down a job." Through the tears in her eyes, it is clear that she has gained much sympathy and respect for this man. I am confident that this encounter has changed her outlook on her disease for life.

10:00 a.m.

The next patient I see is a 49-year-old Hmong-speaking man with epigastric pain who is deaf and mentally delayed. I call for an interpreter and attempt to complete a history and examination. Initial labs and studies are ordered. An hour later, I page surgery because his abdominal ultrasound shows gallstones with a thick gallbladder wall, and his labs show elevated liver transaminase levels, which tells me that he has cholecystitis. I call his family to come in to give surgical consent because of this patient's various limitations.

The patient in room 3 with a chief complaint of flank pain is next on my list. I walk into the room to find an angry couple firing demands and questions at me before I have the chance to introduce myself. "This is our fifth ED visit in the last 2 months, and no one is doing anything!" My patient has a known 8-mm ureteral stone and left-sided *hydronephrosis*. I page the urology PA to decide which further imaging studies are needed because this patient has already had two computed tomographic (CT) scans in the last 8 weeks. I write prescriptions for pain medications and arrange a urology appointment for *nephrostomy* tube placement.

12:00 Noon

I meet my next patient, a 49-year-old man with a history of polysubstance abuse. He complains of pleuritic chest pain, anxiety, and shortness of breath. He has abstained from methamphetamines per a urine toxicology screen, but he continues to smoke one pack of cigarettes, drink 12 beers, and sniff aerosol paint daily. His exam is normal other than metallic paint-stained fingernails. After negative lab results and imaging, I give him educational resource information. He asks for a hot meal and a bus ticket before leaving.

12:45 p.m.

After lunch, I approach a 59-year-old woman who is lying on her side moaning in pain. On physical exam, she has a moist, red, 6- × 4-cm bulge hanging outside her rectum. She has already received pain medications, so I slowly push her prolapsed rectum back in. Her history is significant for schizophrenia. She goes on a vocal tirade that spares no details and tells me her husband is "spiritually raping" her. I write a prescription for stool softeners and pain medication and schedule her for an elective surgery appointment. This patient is now medically cleared, and I page a social worker to evaluate the need to transfer her to a psychiatric facility.

My next encounter is with a 69-year-old aggressive schizophrenic man with suicidal tendencies. He is a tall, thin man, dressed in a blue paper outfit, who is yelling inappropriately, lurching forward in his chair, and attempting to hit people. A police officer stands with me as I examine him and attempt to talk to him. Having little success, I write orders for haloperidol (Haldol) and a benzodiazepine and then transfer him to the behavioral-care unit. He is placed on a 72-hour hold for psychiatric evaluation.

2:00 p.m.

I walk over to another area of the ED where patients with lower-acuity complaints wait. Most have minor issues such as chronic back pain or viral illness or else are waiting for medication refills. These patients should be seeing primary doctors instead, but many are homeless, have no insurance, and harbor little desire to help themselves for the long term. They are looking for a free "quick fix."

One of these patients is a 23-year-old man who has come to request refills on his medications. He had been in a nearly fatal car accident 7 years prior that had caused femur and spinal compression fractures. For reasons unknown to me, he was sentenced to 7 years in prison, during which he was medicated with morphine sulfate. He had been released the previous day. With no insurance and no primary doctor, this patient now faced a new problem of narcotic dependency. I offer him a prescription for 1 week of pain medication and set him up with our financial assistance program.

5:30 p.m.

An attending physician from another zone calls me: "Hey Jessi, I have a *paracentesis* all set up. You should come by." I go over to his patient, perform the procedure, and drain 5 liters of fluid from the cirrhotic patient's belly.

My next patient is a Hispanic man wearing a white shirt splattered with blood. He has a left ear cartilage laceration that occurred because his 19-year-old son threw a glass coffeepot at his head. I ask why his son is still living with him. He responds, "My wife has stage 2 breast cancer and wants him to stay. Every time I try to kick him out, it causes a painful fight with my sick wife." While I'm sewing, I spend 10 to 20 minutes having a personal conversation with a perfect stranger. The ED is a place where patients come during a life crisis, and venting is often a part of the healing process.

My last patient is a cachectic 55-year-old woman with a 4- × 6-cm abscess on her right arm. Twenty years prior, she abused IV drugs. She has lived her life moving from one women's shelter to the next after fleeing abusive relationships. After administering pain medication and explaining the procedure, I begin. I cut a 2-inch incision and drain 20 to 30 mL of purulent fluid from the site. I use forceps to pack the cavity with iodoform gauze, prescribe antibiotics, and instruct her to follow up in 24 hours.

On an average day in the emergency department, I see quite a variety of cases: There are psychiatric, medical, and surgical cases, social dilemmas, substance abuse, system abuse, and primary-care issues. At 7:00 p.m., I give my sign-out to the night-shift PA. Day in and day out, being with people at their time of crisis and poor health authenticates that "good health is the greatest wealth."

Reprinted, with permission, from the *Journal of the American Academy of Physician Assistants*, June 2011.

CHAPTER 8

Working Outside the Box

INTRODUCTION

Generally speaking, physician assistants (PAs) are bright, well-educated, and well-trained individuals in the field of healthcare. PAs can be used in a wide and creative array of ways outside a clinic or hospital environment. This chapter introduces PAs writing about their experiences in unique settings such as administration, anesthesia, and forensics. There are also excerpts about military service, teaching and research, and opportunities outside the United States. If you have a heart for service, a National Health Service Corps scholarship recipient gives tips for the application process, and another inspirational entrepreneur tells his story. Before settling down in a 9 to 5 job in suburbia, read this chapter to expand your horizons.

A DAY IN THE LIFE: NATIONAL HEALTH SERVICE CORPS SCHOLARSHIP RECIPIENT

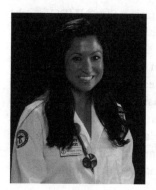

Natasha Ohta, PA-S

There is a Chinese proverb that says, "There are many paths to the top of the mountain, but the view is always the same." I've discovered that within the physician assistant (PA) profession this is especially true because many of us did not set out to become PAs but wonderfully managed to stumble upon the career through various unique experiences. My personal journey to the top of the PA mountain began as a confused biology major at University of California Santa Barbara in an attempt to pursue a career in physical therapy. My hatred of chemistry prompted me to search for a passion elsewhere, landing me in the Global Studies Department, where I became obsessed with culture and travel. After graduating, I thought about joining the Peace Corps, opting instead for a 4-month backpacking adventure through Central and South America, where I stopped briefly in Honduras to volunteer for an American medical brigade that set up temporary clinics in surrounding rural villages. It was there that I witnessed the change brought on by the practice of compassionate medicine, inspiring me to return to my original plan of going into the health professions, but this time with a burning desire to work in an underserved community.

Returning home to the United States, I began the application process for physical therapy programs with the nagging feeling that I was still not quite on the right track. With more research, I simultaneously came across the PA profession and the National Health Service Corps (NHSC), which is a government-funded organization that offers scholarships in exchange for service in federally qualified health professional shortage areas to medical doctors (MDs), doctors of osteopathic medicine (DOs), PAs, nurse midwives, and dentists but not to physical therapists. Feeling an overwhelming sense of purpose, I decided to take a leap of faith, change paths, and pursue a career as a PA so that I could apply for the scholarship. The application process was relatively simple, consisting of two letters of recommendation, three short essays, transcripts, a résumé, and paperwork confirming that I was already accepted into a PA program. It wasn't until a couple of months into the school year, while studying for my first big exam, that I received notice that I was chosen as a NHSC scholarship recipient, thus completing my journey to the top of the mountain.

As an NHSC scholar, I signed a contract stating that NHSC would cover my tuition and provide me with a monthly stipend to cover cost of living and a once-yearly lump sum to cover the cost of books, medical equipment, and other reasonable costs in exchange for a 2-year commitment to serve at a federally qualified health center (FQHC) on completion of my program. These FQHCs consist of underserved rural or urban primary-care clinics, federal prisons, migrant centers, or Indian reservations. Once you receive the scholarship, you must stay in good standing with your program, and if at any point you decide to break your contract with NHSC or are unable to complete your program, you are obligated to pay back three times the amount that NHSC has given you.

In my opinion, one of the biggest misconceptions about the NHSC scholarship is that you have to work where they tell you. Although you are expected to have an open mind and a bit of flexibility as to where you may end up, you are ultimately responsible for finding a job. Although NHSC will place you if you let a certain amount of time lapse after completing your program, the agency strives to retain healthcare workers in under-served communities, so one of its biggest goals is to help you find a job in an area where you are happy and are likely to stay long term. As a scholar, there is an abundance of resources available to help connect you with jobs in the area of your choosing, including two all-expense paid conferences—one at the beginning of your contract and one at the end—where you have the opportunity to meet with the advisors who are there to support you through your NHSC experience, hear stories from past scholars, and even network with potential employers. There are also online resources, includ-ing a job center, where you can research open jobs across the nation and a portal where you have access to continuing medical education (CME) and can watch live webinars on topics of particular interest to those working in underserved area. In the event that you do have to relocate, the scholar-ship pays for you to visit the site prior to moving so that you can see how you would fit within the community, as well as moving expenses one way. If you are interested in seeing what jobs are available in your area or what clinics qualify as FQHCs, you can visit http://nhscjobs.hrsa.gov/external/search/index.seam.

Another way that the NHSC helps to alleviate debt is through the Loan Repayment Program. Recipients of loan payments can receive up to $60,000 toward paying off existing debt for 2 years of full-time service by first securing a job in a loan-repayment-eligible health shortage area, followed by completing the application process. The benefit to the Loan Repayment Program is that there are more clinics that satisfy loan-repayment requirements, whereas clinics that are approved for scholars are those that are considered to be "more underserved." This is deter-mined by a Health Profession Shortage Area (HPSA) score that is given to each FQHC by the federal government based on the number of existing providers in the community, wait time, socioeconomic factors, and so on and ranges from 0 to 26, with 26 being the score given to clinics with the most need. Also, there is less risk involved because NHSC is refunding you for debt that you have already acquired instead of paying your tuition up front. More information on both loan-repayment and scholarship options is available at http://nhsc.hrsa.gov/index.html.

People often ask me why I think I was chosen as a recipient and what they can do to get the scholarship. My answer is that you must have a genuine desire to work in an underserved area long term. The scholarship is not a prize to be won but an opportunity to relieve the burden of debt so that you can pursue jobs in areas where salaries are lower than average. In other words, the desire to work in a low-income area must be there before you apply. If NHSC is something you are considering, my advice is to show a lot of community involvement because the agency is looking not only for great healthcare providers but also leaders who will work hard to empower those within the community to bring about positive change. Although I am still 1 year away from completing my training, I am excited to become part of an existing team—10,000 NHSC healthcare professionals working toward improving access to healthcare by providing high-quality, culturally competent care—and cannot imagine going through this journey in any other way.

A DAY IN THE LIFE: ANESTHESIOLOGY ASSISTANT AND PA

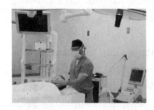

Michael P. Merren, MSM, MMSc, PA-C, AA-C

The field of anesthesia is a practice that has been difficult for physician assistants (PAs) to break into. Currently, in order to practice intraoperative anesthesia as a PA, you must attend an additional anesthesiology assistant (AA) program. This program is similar to PA school with one year of didactic education, one year of clinical rotations, and a national certifying exam on program completion. Once certified, an AA-C can administer anesthesia under the supervision of an anesthesiologist. There are currently eight AA programs in the United States.

After 5 years working as a pulmonary and critical-care PA, I decided to go back to school to attend Emory University's Master of Medical Science Program in Anesthesiology. In my case, tuition was paid because I committed to working at Emory for 3 years after program completion. Becoming an AA-C, as well as a maintaining my PA-C, has allowed me the unique opportunity to practice both intraoperative anesthesia and critical-care medicine. The practice of anesthesia is exceptionally dynamic. There are moments of high stress followed by hours of boredom. The unique challenge of managing patients with multiple comorbidities in the operating room (OR) is what drew my interest to the field of anesthesia.

5:30 a.m.

I change into a set of scrubs and walk into the control center of the OR. In this area, all cases are posted for the day on large monitor screens. The case that I'm assigned is a *coronary artery bypass grafting (CABG)* with an aortic valve replacement in Room 104. Once in my room, I carry out an hour-long room preparation and safety checklist, similar to an airline pilot's preflight checklist. Part of this process includes checking the anesthesia machine, setting up monitors, and preparing all the medications and infusions that may be needed for the case.

6:30 a.m.

The preoperative holding area is where I meet my patient. After introductions, I review his medical history, check his identification band, and ask him to verify the procedure he is going to have, the name of his surgeon, and the time of his last meal. He has an *ejection fraction* of 25 percent with severe aortic stenosis and a left circumflex and right coronary artery lesion that will be repaired using a saphenous vein graft. Communication is vital; next, I go over informed consent regarding the placement of a large-bore peripheral intravenous (IV) arterial line and *pulmonary artery catheter*. I spend the next 30 to 40 minutes placing those lines using sterile technique.

7:30 a.m.

Once in the OR, the circulating nurse again verifies the patient's name, date of birth, procedure, and surgeon. Next, I connect the patient to the monitor, attach the pulmonary artery catheter to a transducer, place defibrillator pads, position the cerebral oximetry montitors, and start to preoxygenate the patient with 100% oxygen. I call the blood bank to make sure that we have blood products available. I next call Dr. Richardson, my supervising anesthesiologist, to let him know that we are ready for induction of anesthesia. Dr. Richardson comes in and supervises as I push the medications to sedate the patient and intubate him. As the anesthetic gas is going through the ventilator, I place a transesophageal *echocardiogram* probe into the patient's esophagus to help assist in monitoring the patient's heart function. Meanwhile, Dr. Richardson leaves the OR and attends to other patients.

8:00 a.m.

The surgeon makes the initial incision, and the 6-hour surgery begins. The patient makes it through the incision without any change in hemodynamics. Now begins the vigilant watchfulness and minor adjustments to *vasopressors* and anesthetic gas levels to help maintain hemodynamics throughout the case.

10:00 a.m.

The chest is open, and the patient has been given a large dose of heparin to *anticoagulate* him, and we go onto *cardiopulmonary bypass (CPB)* and cool the patient down to 32°C. During this time, my job is to help maintain adequate mean arterial pressure, monitor *arterial blood* gas parameters, monitor cerebral oxygen values, provide adequate neuromuscular relaxation, and monitor urine output.

10:30 a.m.

Dr. Richardson comes back to give me a 15-minute break. I go down to the anesthesia lounge to eat a snack and catch up with colleagues.

12:00 Noon

The patient has been on CPB for 2 hours now. I infuse 2 units of fresh-frozen *plasma* to help decrease the chance of postoperative coagulopathy. The latest blood gas determination reveals good oxygenation and ventilation, but the patient's *hematocrit* is down to 19. I discuss this with the surgeon, and we decide to give 2 units of packed red blood cells as well.

12:30 p.m.

One of my anesthesia PA colleagues, Phil, comes in to give me a 30-minute lunch break.

1:00 p.m.

Done with lunch, I come into the OR to find that we are getting ready for the patient to start being weaned from CPB. I start a milrinone drip in anticipation of needing support due to the patient's poor baseline heart function. I call the blood bank to have 4 units of blood brought up in anticipation of post-CPB anemia. After warming, the heart is still not attempting to beat well on its own, so we charge the internal defibrillator paddles and shock the heart. The heart then starts beating and contracting on its own. I call Dr. Richardson to perform a transesophageal echocardiogram to make sure that all the air is out of the heart as it is pumping while still on CPB. The heart is deaired, and then we start to lower the support from the CPB until the heart is doing all the work on its own with some pharmacologic assistance.

1:30 p.m.

I am busily monitoring heart function and transfusing the patient with fresh-frozen plasma, packed red blood cells, and cryoprecipitate to correct the patient's coagulopathy. Finally, the bleeding and coagulopathy improve, and the surgeons start closing the chest.

2:30 p.m.

I call up to the cardiothoracic intensive-care unit (CICU) to give a report on the patient. Before transport from the OR to the CICU, I organize my lines so that they do not get tangled or, worse, pulled out during transport.

3:00 p.m.

Once in the CICU, I ensure that my patient is stable, and I communicate with the CICU nurse. Afterwards, I return to the OR to clean up all the medications used and replace the monitors. The next half hour is spent re-setting up the OR in case an emergency surgery is necessary during the night shift.

5:00 p.m.

I check the schedule for the next day to find out what case I have been assigned to. I read about the patient's past medical history on the computer to be better prepared. It has been a long and productive day in the OR. Unlike other medical practices, my day may only involve one or two patients in a 12-hour period. Now it's time to head home and enjoy some time with my wife and two boys.

The practice of anesthesia integrates many different medical specialties wrapped into one. I enjoy starting a new adventure with every patient I have. You never know how a patient is going to respond initially to anesthesia or surgery, so you are the main person responsible for making sure that the whole patient is being taken care of. I encourage any PAs who are interested in this field to pursue it because each year there are more and more practices opening their doors and looking for anesthesia assistants to become part of their team.

A DAY IN THE LIFE: FORENSICS

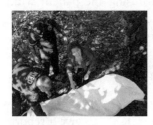

Louise Capellupo, MS, PA-C, D-ABMDI

In 2002, I was hired as a medicolegal death investigator, and in the job I spent my time at Ground Zero following the World Trade Center disaster. I was closely involved with the identification process of approximately 20,000 body parts as I worked with medical examiners, anthropologists, forensic odontologists, and DNA scientists. We reviewed missing persons' data received from the victims' family members and then requested items that belonged to the victims such as a toothbrush, hairbrush, or clothing. When a positive DNA match was confirmed, we communicated with family members. To this day, 59 percent of the victims have been identified.

As a medicolegal investigator, my responsibilities are to respond to all manner of reported deaths regardless of complexity. This work is coordinated with members of the New York Police Department (NYPD) Crime Scene Unit when indicated. My duties are to photograph and examine the body at the scene; categorize and transport potential evidence; interview family members, physicians, and witnesses; and obtain positive identification and a signed affidavit. When necessary, these duties also can include identification through dental records, x-rays, fingerprints, and circumstantial information. My responsibilities also include collection of exemplar evidence from suspects, defendants, victims, and victim-associated persons. This may be blood, head or pubic hair, and buccal swabs at the request of district attorney's office or court order.

I have been involved in criminal investigations, including domestic abuse, child abuse, homicides by gunfire, stabbing, gunshot wounds prior to burning, strangulation, and head trauma. I have investigated scenes where various body parts were found in bags or suitcases in parks, basements, abandoned houses, closets, garbage trucks, and alleys and embedded in cement. I also have had to respond to demolition and construction sites where a backhoe operator discovered "unknown" bones.

One needs to be relatively fit to stand on a bed and pull a 300-pound man onto his abdomen, to pull a floater from the river onto a rocky embankment, to climb a ladder into a subceiling after an electrician has electrocuted himself, and to crawl into the wheel well of an inbound jumbo jet after a frozen stowaway is discovered by the maintenance crew. This is not a job for the faint of heart.

Death investigation and its association with forensic science is a field that employs very few PAs. It makes sense that our foundation and training in observation and external examination can be applied to settings outside the typical hospital or physician's office. We provide the link between the death scene and the autopsy so that the medical examiner has as much information as possible to determine the cause and manner of death. This area of work requires a blend of intestinal fortitude and compassion. Notwithstanding, it highlights the versatility of a physician assistant (PA) education whereby the basics of a good physical exam can be applied to the dead as well as the living.

Here is an example of a day in the life:

9:00 a.m.

Desk phone rings. "Hi officer, this is Investigator Capellupo. What do we have?"

"A DOA [dead on arrival]."

I pull up the Notice of Death on the computer. "So it's a 51-year-old man. What were the circumstances of him being found?"

"He lived alone. The building superintendent hadn't seen him for about 2 weeks. He wasn't answering his door, so the super used the spare key to get in. He found the body and called 911."

"Secured premises?"

"Affirmative."

"Where is he in the apartment?"

"Face up on the living room floor. But he's a bit of a pack rat, and he is on top of a lot of stuff."

"Did EMS work on him?"

"No, they said he's been gone a while—there are flies and maggots around his head, and the smell is pretty bad."

"Any signs of drugs or alcohol?"

"Yeah, it looks like he was a bit of a drinker. Four or five empty bottles of vodka in the kitchen, plus a few in the bedroom. I don't see any drugs, but there is so much stuff here."

"So no signs of forced entry? Any suspicious circumstances?"

"The detectives were here and don't think there is anything unusual. But they will come back if you need them."

"Does he have family to provide information about his past medical history?"

"We're trying to contact a brother in New Jersey."

"Ok, I'll be there within the hour."

9:30 a.m.

I arrive at the apartment building, photograph the outside, and press the buzzer. No answer after several attempts. Then I realize that if the body is decomposed and stinky, the officer will probably be sitting in the hallway and won't hear the buzzer.

Just as I am about to press the neighbor's buzzer, a resident approaches the front door and sees my jacket that reads, "NYC Office of Chief Medical Examiner." She lets me in but with nervous curiosity asks, "Is someone dead?"

I go to the seventh floor, making note of the type of building and how many floors in total. I step out of the elevator, and the stench hits me. The police officer, sitting on a chair in the hallway, is happy to see me. He hands me the toe tag to sign.

I stand at the doorway of the decedent's apartment and think, "Oh no . . . a decomposed hoarder." Photographing the scene, I scramble like a mountain goat over piles of newspapers, clothes, bike parts, plastic bags, and empty cereal boxes. I find the body lying on cardboard cartons, books, plastic cups, tattered Christmas decorations, and newspapers. And then I see a thin man wearing only a shirt. The only sign of movement is the sea of maggots traveling in and out of his eyes, nose, and mouth. The stench is profound—a density in the air.

Before I turn my "patient" prone, I look around the apartment for any medications, hospital bills, or doctors' or dentists' cards? I go into the bedroom, bathroom, and kitchen. Did he have esophageal *varices* and succumb to a massive gastrointestinal (GI) bleed? Any blood on the floor or in the toilet bowl? On paper towels in the kitchen? Any drugs or associated paraphernalia?

I lift his head and feel for a deformity. No bullet holes. I look to see if there are any other signs of obvious trauma. I flip him over. No knife in his back and no blood spatter on the walls or ceiling. My physical exam is limited, however, due to the degree of decomposition. Normally, I would look for *petechial hemorrhages* in the eyes, areas of *ecchymosis* to the neck and beyond, inner lip abrasions or lacerations, surgical scars, physical deformities, and tattoos for identification purposes, determine the degree of lividity and rigor mortis, and take a rectal temperature—all part of the physical exam on a fresh body.

10:25 a.m.

I call for the morgue van to pick him up, and I leave the building, wondering what the autopsy will show. Did he have significant liver disease from his chronic alcohol abuse, signs of long-standing hypertension, coronary artery disease, or a *subdural hematoma* from a fall in a drunken *stupor*? Does he have children who care about him? Does he have a loving family who will make funeral arrangements and give him a proper burial?

11:45 a.m.

Back at the office, I start to download my photos and begin typing up the report. Another call. This time from an emergency room (ER) attending at a local teaching hospital, wanting to discuss a case.

"A 68 year old obese man with a history of hypertension, hypercholesterolemia, and diabetes. Got up out of bed to go to the bathroom this morning. His wife heard a thud and found him on the bathroom floor. She attempted cardiopulmonary resuscitation (CPR). Emergency Medical Services (EMS) arrived, found him in asystole, and initiated the Advanced

Cardiac Life Support (ACLS) protocol. He was intubated in the field and transported here, still in cardiac arrest. He got epinephrine and *vasopressin*; we worked on him for another 15 minutes and then pronounced him dead at 10:17 hours. Downtime was about 45 minutes. His wife said he was taking medication for his blood pressure, and the diabetes was diet-controlled. But she indicated that he was not very compliant."

"Any signs of trauma to the body?"

"No."

"Do you suspect any illicit drugs or alcohol contributed to his death?"

"No."

"Are you comfortable signing the death certificate?"

"Yes, I was going to sign it as 'hypertensive cardiovascular disease' with 'diabetes mellitus' as a contributing condition."

"Yes, that's fine. If the family wants an autopsy, your hospital can perform it. This is not a medical examiner's case. My name is Investigator Capellupo. Thanks, doctor. Have a nice day."

I continue writing up my investigative report on the alcoholic hoarder and grab a bite to eat.

1:56 p.m.

"Capellupo, we have another case for you, out of the 121st Precinct. An apparent shooting, and an officer is on the line, I'll transfer him."

"Hi officer, what do we have?"

"A 28-year-old in the garage of a house. A neighbor heard some arguing. Several shots were fired, and then two unknown individuals were seen running up the street."

"Is Crime Scene on their way?"

"Yeah, I'll call you when they have finished processing the scene."

3:45 p.m.

I arrive at the scene and gain access through the cordoned off perimeter, marked by that familiar yellow tape. I gather whatever information is available from the catching detective; however, it's sketchy at best. We are in a quiet residential neighborhood, but it's a "no-one knows nothin' . . ." situation. Apparently, the decedent lived in the garage, and his mother lived upstairs. Crime scene detectives have taken their pictures and are now ready for me to examine the body.

On the floor of this converted garage is a well-built, muscular young man in a left lateral recumbent position. The left side of his face is resting in a pool of blood, and he is wearing baggy jeans and a blood-soaked T-shirt with a skull pattern. I take my photos of the surroundings and the lifeless body, stepping with trepidation across puddles of pungent blood. One can't be leaving footprints at the crime scene. Relatives are arriving outside the house. They are screaming, sobbing, and audibly grieving, being kept away from the immediate vicinity by NYPD officers. I cannot interact with the family. The consequences would be too chaotic. I must concentrate on what I see, describe the scene, and identify the wounds. Any weapons? Bullet casings? Drugs? What happened here?

Multiple wounds to the chest, back, and head. No, I cannot determine which are entrance and which are exit wounds here. That will be done at autopsy. I don't want the detectives hanging their hats on ". . . an entrance wound here, so therefore the shooter was standing there." This is rule number one that investigators learn early in their on-the-job training.

I find a wallet in his jeans with a tentative identification. There is over $1,600 in $100 bills. I give the wallet containing the money to the vouchering police officer, and he signs the personal property paperwork. I look around for drugs, but the area is in disarray—overturned furniture and signs of a struggle. I call for the morgue van and leave the scene. Not a lot to do here because the NYPD Crime Scene detectives remain at the location to continue their evidence collection and scene investigation.

On the way back to the office, I receive a call about some unknown bones found at the edge of a pond. The responding police officer reported that a passerby collecting cans and bottles in this remote swamp found seven bones, all approximately 5 to 6 inches long. At the scene, I lay them on a log with a ruler and appreciate that they are old and intact. "Could this be a child?" the detective inquires?

"Unlikely," I reply. "They look like animal bones, maybe a dog?" I photograph them and e-mail my pictures to the anthropologist on duty. A quick reply states, "Nonhuman."

5:00 p.m.

Back at the office, I type my reports about the gunshot victim and the partial remains of someone's pet. Today I have tried to gather multiple pieces of multiple puzzles, calling on my years of experience as an emergency medicine physician assistant (PA). I don't need a stethoscope, I don't carry a gun, I don't wear high heels, I don't look under microscopes, and I don't perform autopsies. The tools of my trade are a camera, a flashlight, latex gloves, and a rectal thermometer. I feel sad for the victims. I wonder about the lives they have led and how their families will cope with the news of their death. It doesn't matter whether the deceased lived in a homeless encampment in the woods or in a beautiful upscale Manhattan home. They all are people who will not experience another day. I have touched and examined the empty shell that they once lived in.

I may not be treating patients in a hospital, but all these DOAs are my patients. Instead of working with nurses and doctors, I am working with police officers and detectives. I do my best to provide the results of my investigation to the medical examiner who will perform the autopsy the next day and who will ultimately determine the cause and manner of death. I must be objective, observant, unbiased, nonjudgmental, and detached but empathetic.

As a PA, I feel privileged that I have this unique opportunity to use my clinical skills in the field of forensic investigations. After a day spent on the darker side of life, I go home and give my kids that extra hug. Through death, one learns to appreciate life.

A DAY IN THE LIFE: ADMINISTRATION

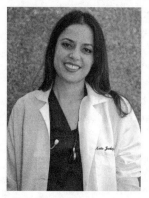

Azita Javdanfar, MS, PA-C

Immediately after physician assistant (PA) school, I was fortunate enough to get a position in one of the largest county emergency departments (EDs) in the western United States. The field of emergency medicine drew me in because of its fast pace, interesting patient cases, and 12-hour shift schedule. However, the most rewarding aspect is the ability to take care of the underserved patient population. The county hospital and outpatient clinics are the only accessible routes of healthcare for these patients, many with diagnoses such as cancer, heart failure, and diabetes. Having a significant impact on another individual's life is the most exciting part of being a PA.

After 2 years as a clinical ED PA, an opening for an administrative position came up within the ED. This position was designed for a PA or nurse practitioner to assist with various projects that focus on improving patient flow and subsequently patient care. I was attracted to the uniqueness of the position because I could help patients on a macroscopic level. A sample of my day is as follows:

7:30 a.m.

I arrive at my office and generate the weekly data-report sheet to present in the upcoming morning meeting. The report contains statistics on patient care, such as number of patients seen in the last week, wait times, and patient disposition times. It is generated for analysis and consideration of improving patient care.

8:30 a.m.

The clinical directors' meeting begins; the attendees include the ED medical directors, nursing supervisors, and various other ED heads (such as the directors of the psychiatric ED and pediatrics ED and quality improvement supervisors). I stand and present the results of the weekly data report. At the meeting, other ED issues at hand are discussed, and I have the opportunity to contribute ideas for improving patient flow.

10:30 a.m.

After the meeting, I go to the newly designed patient-care area of our ED. This modified fast-track area is an ED project in the making. It was proposed as an idea to supplement the current fast-track area to treat patients of moderate acuity who are too complicated for the current fast-track area. I am assigned to oversee this area and help to ensure its proper functioning and flow. Today I will be training a new group of nursing attendants (NAs) to work in the area. The NAs are responsible for ensuring that the booths are filled with patients and for helping the nurses with various issues. I teach the NAs how to use our electronic medical records system to allow them to bring patients from the waiting room to be seen by a medical provider. I also make sure that the area is stocked with appropriate supplies, including the ED ultrasound machine. If I notice that a supply is missing, I quickly find a replacement. So far, the area is working well to ensure quicker patient care. Resting assured that there are no active issues, I can now take my lunch break.

1:00 p.m.

After lunch, I review charts from yesterday's patients who presented to the ED but left without being seen. Most patients leave without evaluation by a physician secondary to long wait times in an overwhelmed county system. I read the charts and call the patients one by one, encouraging them to return to the ED for a complete evaluation. One example case is a 65-year-old woman who presented with flulike symptoms, had a chest x-ray ordered by the triage nurse, and left after a long wait before receiving the results. The x-ray shows evidence of consolidation in the left lower lung base consistent with pneumonia. I share this information with the patient over the phone, and when she returns to the ED 30 minutes later, I guide her to the appropriate area to receive her antibiotics.

3:30 p.m.

I divert my attention to a new project—designing and creating an internal ED website. It is intended to serve as a resource for ED staff. I work to collect material such as the hospital antibiogram, the antibiotic list from the pharmacy, various policies, electronic versions of the various forms we use in the ED, and the ED specialty consult list. Once all the new material is added, I show it to the medical director. He agrees that the website is ready to launch.

Working as an administrative PA is unique. It is a quiet, slow-paced job with normal weekday hours. It is much different than the chaotic nature of being a clinical ED PA, which requires a mixture of night shifts, midafternoon shifts, weekends, and holidays. Clinical ED PAs historically have a reputation for frequent burnout due to the ever-changing schedule and the demands of the actual workday—the constant sense of urgency and multitasking. This temporary change in the role of administration allows me to avoid burnout, gain perspective, and care for patients on a grand scale. And I am still doing what matters most, making a difference in patients' lives.

A DAY IN THE LIFE: AN INSPIRATIONAL ENTREPRENEUR

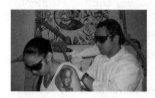

Pedro Gonzalez, PA-C

The physician assistant (PA) profession was foreign to me, growing up as I did in the streets of East Los Angeles. In those days, I would have never guessed the enormous possibilities in this great career. The profession has given me the knowledge and experience to deal with the harsh realities of East LA and to help people there in ways I never would have thought possible. I've been very fortunate to find work that allows me to contribute to the health of individual patients and to the greater health of the community.

Recently, I worked with three partners to establish a bakery, Mi Vida—My Life, that offers healthy products to help prevent diabetes, obesity, hypertension, and hyperlipidemia. We have a website (www.mividamylife.com) and a retail store in Lynwood, CA. We have customers such as Bristol Farms Deli Department (California), The Delivery Zone/Sunfare.com (Arizona, California), and Natural Slim (Puerto Rico). We are also approved vendors for the Obesity Prevention Program at the Los Angeles Unified School District. The retail store sells an array of bread loaves, tortillas, cookies, and Mexican sweet bread. It's been a humbling experience for our bakery to receive national media attention from several television stations and newspapers.

The bakery also houses the Homeboy Industries bakery training program, where former gang members work side by side with regular workers and with each other to gain skills to help them redirect their lives. Nationally recognized by First Lady Laura Bush, Homeboy Industries (www.homeboy-industries.org) is an employment-referral center and economic-development program that assists 1,000 people a month. "Nothing stops a bullet like a job" is its guiding principle.

The principles of the PA profession include caring for the underserved and helping the less fortunate. I try to do this by giving back to those from my childhood community and by telling my story to inspire others to do the same. I believe that what I do is much needed by people who deserve a second chance at life and who are "a whole lot more than the worst thing they've ever done."

7:00 a.m. (Monday, Friday)

On Monday and Friday mornings I'm at the bakery to oversee its management and to hold group talks with the regular employees and the Homeboy bakers to foster open communication. These talks help the Homeboy bakers, many of whom have been incarcerated, make the transition from highly regulated prison life to life on the outside with its flexible boundaries. I also make follow-up calls to clients and schedule meetings. Some bakery clients are walk-in customers whose health we monitor. Most thank us for producing great products that have helped them control their health problems. We schedule monthly group meetings for members of the community, where we discuss a variety of diseases. These meetings are fun, and they let me educate the community in a relaxed atmosphere with no stethoscope draped around my neck. We also were honored with invitations from the American Heart Association Health Partners program and the Latino Diabetes Association to present educational sessions as well.

11:00 a.m. to 5:00 p.m. (Monday, Friday)

On Mondays and Fridays I also work in a pediatrics practice, where my day is full of physical exams and upper respiratory infections. Among my favorite parts are the well-child visits from kids 2 weeks to 1 year old, and I enjoy calming parents' worries about their children's progress. Then it's off to administer vaccinations and watch an adorable baby's face become a siren of crying. Last week I sutured a child's lacerated forearm after a skateboard accident. To my surprise, he was very happy about the situation. When I asked him why, he said, "Now I don't have to do chores for 2 or 3 weeks." This made me laugh.

9:00 a.m. to 12:30 p.m. (Tuesday, Wednesday, Thursday)

These mornings I work in a community-based internal medicine/family practice clinic where many of the patients are geriatric, and most are Latino or Asian. I'm the only Spanish-speaking clinician at this clinic, which attends to approximately 55 patients a day. Two physicians and I treat patients with a variety of diseases from diabetes to cancer. I do 95 percent of the clinical work and act as a translator when needed, under the guidance of my medical director. At times, I talk with my patients about quality of life, and it's then that I reflect on my own life and health. From time to time, I listen to my own heart and lungs to make sure that I am ticking and breathing correctly! I get a kick out of trying to communicate in different languages, and in response, I often get an appreciative pat on my cheek or shoulder, a bow, or a heavily accented, "Thank you."

1:30 to 6:00 p.m. (Wednesday, Thursday)

On Wednesday and Thursday afternoons I work at Homeboy Industries' Ya 'Stuvo (That's Enough) Tattoo Removal Program in East Los Angeles. I began there as a volunteer, but now I'm a senior staff person, and part of what I do is train other clinicians in tattoo removal. The program provides accessible, no-cost tattoo-removal services to former gang members of all races who enroll voluntarily. Tattoos of the kind we work on are stigmatizing and prevent those who have them from getting and keeping jobs and from integrating socially in other ways. We give priority to those with gang tattoos visible on the face, head, neck, or fingers and to those with children. A typical day is filled with approximately 20 patients, about a third female.

A typical treatment session goes like this: The patient walks in looking concerned, and 95 percent of the time the first question is, "Does it hurt?" I explain the procedure, the complications, and the results that can be realistically expected with our Palomar Q-YAG 5 laser. We prep using universal precautions and begin the treatment with a test shot from the laser. Many patients can withstand the burning feeling, but if the pain is intolerable, we offer an anesthetic cream at no cost to the patient. On average, six to eight treatments per tattoo are required, and even though treatments are painful, virtually 100 percent of patients complete the process.

Sometimes reporters, college students, or community activists from all over the world stop by to learn about and from Homeboy Industries. On occasion, patients give these visitors permission to observe the treatment. Visitors have described the experience as "surreal, like something out of *National Geographic*."

After treatment, the patient scrutinizes the results in the mirror, usually with some astonishment. We apply antibiotic ointment, dress the area with gauze, and provide preprinted after-care instructions. To date, I have performed more than 1,000 treatments that would have cost patients $250,000 if they had had to pay. My supervising physician meets with me once a week to see how treatments are progressing.

I try also to expand the program by searching for new clinicians to volunteer. We recently received a $50,000 donation to buy a second laser machine, and we've increased our waiting list to approximately 2,000 people. If you're ever in the area and would like a tour or have time to volunteer, please stop by. Our phone number is (323) 526-1254.

I always wanted to come back to the inner city where I was born and raised and provide culturally sensitive healthcare. Becoming a PA has allowed me to make my dreams a reality in more ways than one. God bless the profession for the gifts it has given me, professionally, physically, and spiritually.

Pedro Gonzalez is a PA and an entrepreneur in Los Angeles, CA. He has indicated no relationships to disclose relating to the content of this piece.

Reprinted, with permission, from the *Journal of the American Academy of Physician Assistants*, August 2006.

PA OPPORTUNITIES OUTSIDE THE U.S.

A DAY IN THE LIFE: VOLUNTEERING IN RWANDA

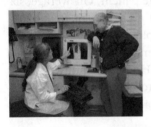

Rebecca Tinsman, RPA-C

I'm volunteering for a month at the WE-ACTx Clinic, Kigali, Rwanda. This all came about when one of the clinic founders, Dr. Kathy Anastos, spoke at our HIV rounds. Kathy talked about her clinic in Rwanda, founded when she and Anne-Christine D'adesky, an HIV activist and Pulitzer-nominated writer, wanted to help the HIV-infected people of Rwanda after the 1994 genocide. More than 250,000 Tutsi women were raped by Hutu men during the 100 days of genocide. Today, many of the women infected with HIV during the genocide have AIDS and are in need of experienced medical care. Rwanda is now one of the most stable countries in Africa, but it is still struggling to meet the needs of the sick. When capable foreign aid is offered, it is often accepted.

7:00 a.m.

I leave the house in the Kiyovu section of Kigali for the 25-minute walk to the clinic. The walk is all uphill and down and around. "Around" because President Kagame's compound extends to the most direct route, and the road is blocked and heavily guarded. "Uphill and down" because Rwanda is known as "the land of one thousand hills" for good reason. If you should mention his country's sobriquet to a Rwandan, he will tell you that whoever was counting the hills missed a few.

WE-ACTx is on one of the main streets in Kigali, not far from the embassies and big nongovernment organization (NGO) offices. The clinic is on the second floor of a new building and has a wide balcony overlooking the street. The women who come to the clinic for their semiannual visits often sit there and talk while they eat the breakfast that the clinic provides. Some of the women walk for hours to get their care. Others take minibuses, which are actually vans into which 16 to 20 people are crammed. The buses cost about 75 cents. Nothing to you and me, but that's nearly the average daily income in Rwanda!

I get to the clinic and climb the steep stairs. The women in the waiting room are singing hymns. Ambient clinic and street noises disappear behind their voices. Before setting up the exam room with Bosco, the Rwandan nurse I work with, I go to the bathroom. No water today. The water comes via an artesian system, and the water table is too low now. Someone brings up water in a 5-gallon plastic jug. That water is used to flush the toilet, to wash hands, and to hand wash the clinic laundry.

WE-ACTx stands for Women's Equity in Access to Care and Treatment (www.we-actx.org). WE-ACTx has two parts: the RWISA study clinic and the ambulatory HIV clinic. We are working on the RWISA study—the Rwanda Women's Inter-Association Study, a sister to the stateside Women's Interagency HIV Study (WIHS). In addition to examining the women, we attempt to document any corporal changes HIV may effect. The study at WE-ACTx has 800 HIV-positive women and 200 HIV-negative control individuals. HIV infection is generally not treated in Rwanda until the CD4 cell count drops below $200/\mu L$ or the patient suffers an opportunistic infection. At that point, antiretroviral therapy is usually instituted. At WE-ACTx, most of the women I meet are on a fixed-dose regimen containing nevirapine (Viramune).

8:00 a.m. to Noon

Bosco and I call in the first woman we are to see. *Phlebotomy* for fasting labs is the first order of business in the morning. The labs are the usual—CD4 cell count, viral load, complete blood count (CBC), urinalysis, and comprehensive panel. Just as I am ready to insert my butterfly into my first patient's vein, the electricity goes out, as it does nearly every day, and we are thrown into near darkness. Bosco puts a miner's lamp on my head, and I resume work. We draw blood from six women, and after they eat, we call them back for their exams.

As I put the blood pressure cuff around one woman's arm, she says something to Bosco in Kinyarwanda. Bosco laughs and tells me, "She says her pressure will be high because she has never been touched by a *muzungu* (white person) before." That possibility has never occurred to me. I find that whites, especially outside Kigali, are a rarity and a source of much interest. No matter where I walk, I hear "*Muzungu! Muzungu!*" inevitably followed by the patter of running feet as children excitedly run to look at me and to touch me if possible. I have long, bright-red hair, which increases my "museum specimen" quotient exponentially. By the end of my stay in Rwanda, I am used to having my hair pulled—not as a prank, but out of curiosity. Most Rwandans have never seen or felt anything like it. They are fascinated.

Walking alone through a village in the Nyungwe National Forest, I don't get more than 50 yards before I have about 20 children walking with me. The brave ones grab my hands and actually fight over who gets to touch me as we walk. I look at them, shake a finger, and say, "No fighting!" They don't understand the words, but they definitely get the message because the rest of the walk is quiet, albeit weird. I feel like the Pied Piper of Hamelin.

The women Bosco and I see at the RWISA clinic all get very basic exams, which include breast and pelvic exams. We do *Pap smears* and cervical lavages. It is not routine for women to have pelvic exams in Rwanda, and right now, even if Pap smears were routine, there are few doctors to treat any abnormalities. While I am in Kigali, a WE-ACTx patient dies of cervical cancer because there was no treatment available to her when it was detected.

Many of my patients have scars, physical as well as emotional, from the genocide. I see an arm missing a hand, machete hash marks across a chest and abdomen, and slash wounds across faces. One woman has a prosthetic leg, which, incongruously, is white. In the streets I see legless teenage boys perched on hand-operated tricycles. I see another boy whose legs were amputated at the top of the thigh. He puts oven mitts on his hands and gets around by leapfrogging through the streets of Kigali. A man with one leg pole vaults from place to place. The genocide is still visible everywhere you look in Rwanda.

If any of the RWISA women are sick, they are referred immediately to the WE-ACTx side of the clinic to be treated by Rwandan doctors. During my stay, I see malaria, tuberculosis, and odd, bullous insect-bite lesions. I see an inordinately high number of breast disorders—deformities as well as masses. One woman I examine has a machete scar on one breast that is still infected 12 years after the fact!

12:00 Noon

Lunchtime. Lunch is usually goat meat samosas and tea, followed by a walk to the market and shops or just a rest on the balcony watching the people below go about their daily business.

1:00 to 5:00 p.m.

No patients in the afternoon. I usually work on the talk I give to the nurses each Friday. I keep it short and relevant—about how the different antiretroviral classes work, for instance, or about sexually transmitted diseases. I hire a translator and make slides. The nurses are really curious and want to learn, but they don't have the resources to research on their own. Books are scarce, clinic computers are rarely free, and the computer café downstairs is expensive.

One afternoon I went to the clinic's food program distribution center. There, all the women in the RWISA study are given 50-pound bags of corn meal fortified with soy protein, out of which they make a thick porridge. Each month they receive a bag. For some families this grain is the only source of food they have, other than the food they can grow for themselves. In a drought, it may be the only food period.

At the center, there is a small shop where widows whose husbands were killed in the genocide and one widower work together to make pretty aprons and dolls in traditional Rwandan dress. They sell these items, which gives them a reasonable income. More important than the income, however, the shop applies President Kagame's plan for reconciliation by employing both Hutu and Tutsi survivors—who now call themselves, simply, Rwandans.

Today I go to Icyzuzo to teach future HIV health educators about viral replication and where antiretroviral agents interfere with that process. There are about 50 teenagers in the classroom. They look at me so intently that I am disconcerted for a while, but eventually I relax. I have a great translator, a college student who is studying medicine at the state university in Butare. Together we manage to present the lecture intelligibly, I think. Afterwards, the questions are just astounding: Is it true that all HIV-positive people in America are isolated from the rest of the population to prevent the spread of HIV? Why do T cells get higher in the United States and stay there compared with Rwanda? Why is the spread of HIV so much higher in sub-Saharan Africa than in the United States?

5:00 p.m.

It's the end of my work day. I take a packed minibus from Icyzuzo to the center of Kigali and walk the rest of the way back, uphill and down and around, to my digs on the outskirts of town.

Rebecca Tinsman works at St. Vincent's HIV Center in Greenwich Village, NY. She has indicated no relationships to disclose relating to the content of this piece.

Reprinted, with permission, from the *Journal of the American Academy of Physician Assistants*, March 2009.

A DAY IN THE LIFE: MISSIONARY IN SUDAN

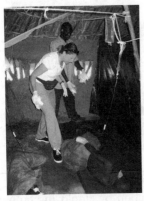

Catherine Hoelzer, MPH, PA-C

6:30 a.m.

The sun is blazing, and the sky is clear. It's going to be a hot day here where I work with a nongovernment organization (NGO) called Christian Mission Aid (CMA) in the upper Nile region of southern Sudan. It has suffered from the longest running civil war in African history, which just came to an end in January 2005. War continues to plague the nation of Sudan in Darfur, but here in the southeastern region of southern Sudan the main troubles are interclan conflicts and militias in the south being armed by the northern government to disrupt the peace process.

We work in four regions providing healthcare and other services to underserved and difficult-to-access communities. We employ locally trained Sudanese community health workers (CHWs) and nurses to work in the primary healthcare clinics. My husband and I joined CMA as missionaries, and we love our work. Although I also loved working in the states as a physician assistant (PA), mainly in internal medicine and urgent care, I knew that I would eventually use my knowledge and training to serve in developing nations, especially in regions that have suffered from war and disaster. In the past, I have worked in other war-torn countries, such as Northern Iraq, Bosnia, Afghanistan, and Chad, and I have always enjoyed being able to help those who have so little.

9:00 a.m.

This morning I'm supervising the CHWs in the maternal child health clinic. The majority of the patients we see in the first hour are children with watery diarrhea—not uncommon in a region where there are only one or two wells. Much of the population gets its water directly from the swamp that surrounds the region we work in.

10:00 a.m.

A young mother brings in her 1-year-old child with complaints of bumps on his head that won't go away. Her husband has been buying penicillin from the local "healer," and when the child gets the injections, he does a bit better. He has two fairly large, hard, cystic-type lesions at the base of his left mastoid and multiple smaller, boggy, crusted lesions on the top of his head. The CHW confers with me because he is not quite sure how to diagnose this child's illness. I have seen these lesions before. The ones on top of the head are usually caused by poor hygiene or mosquito bites that become secondarily infected. I'm a bit more concerned about the other two cystic lesions because they may be TB *adenitis*, which is common here. I tell our CHW to please have the mother come back if the lesions have not resolved after the child finishes the course of penicillin. We might have to refer the child to the County Hospital in Old Fangak, which is a 2-day journey by foot because we have no roads here and no vehicles.

11:00 a.m.

A nurse wants me to see a 3-week-old child whom she suspects is having febrile *convulsions* from neonatal *sepsis*. When I get to the ward, I notice that the child looks more like he is in *spasm* than in convulsions. I ask the mother if she has ever been immunized against tetanus. She has not, so I next ask if she gave birth alone or with the assistance of a trained traditional birth attendant. She gave birth alone and cut the umbilical cord with some grass. Now I'm quite sure the child has neonatal tetanus and realize we must get an intravenous (IV) line in him and begin all the proper medications. We also must try to keep the child in a quiet environment. All this is very difficult when you have several family members in the one-room ward, chickens and dogs running in and out, and other children laughing and crying. I try to explain to our CHWs that we have to get this room quiet somehow. As I walk away, I hear the noise in the room begin to grow. I pray that God will put his hand on that child and heal him. This is often the only hope we have.

12:00 Noon

A mother tells us that her child has been coughing for 2 months. She came to the clinic last month and was given some amoxicillin for a respiratory tract infection. However, as the child has been waiting to be seen, I have not observed him coughing at all. As we get the history from the mother, we learn that the child's illness started off as a common cold, and then about 2 weeks later he started having bouts of coughing that would end with vomiting. When I find out that the child has never been immunized, I realize he is suffering from *whooping cough*. The treatment for this is erythromycin, which is effective only when the child is in the *catarrhal* phase. I prescribe the medication anyway because it also can help decrease the spread of the disease. This is important in a region where so few have been vaccinated.

12:45 p.m.

We have finished seeing patients, and now it is time for lunch, but I'm called to the inpatient department to evaluate a difficult case. A man brought in from a village 2 hours away is in severe respiratory distress. He has a history of asthma and now is in status asthmaticus. He was put on an IV drip and given hydrocortisone, aminophylline, and salbutamol. We don't have oxygen or nebulizers here, so this is all we can provide. When I see him, he is sitting tripod, cannot speak, and is coughing up large mucous plugs with much difficulty. I advise that we give some *adrenaline* if he doesn't improve. As I leave, I think of all the equipment I used to have available to me when I worked in the United States. There is so little here, yet the equipment would be useless because we don't even have electricity.

4:00 p.m.

The heat is beginning to subside, and we make rounds in the inpatient wards. I see that our man in status asthmaticus has improved slightly and can now speak a bit. We have a variety of other patients in the ward who are suffering from severe gastroenteritis or *hemorrhaging* from first-trimester miscarriages. I'm saddened by the number of children who suffer from diseases that could be so easily prevented by simple measures such as immunizations, clean water, and using insecticide-treated bed nets.

5:30 p.m.

I go back to the children's ward to check on the child with neonatal tetanus. He's still in spasm and is getting too much stimuli. I try to encourage the mother again to keep the baby covered and to let him rest. While in the clinic, I'm asked to help with a few of the patients. One is a 7-year-old girl who broke her arm falling out of a tree. She has an open compound fracture that was put back in place by the CHW and then put in a crude splint. The child's father took his daughter to the traditional healer after she fractured her forearm, and the healer "cut" her, a common practice here. They cut a small incision to release the "bad blood." Once the blood is let, they put in some traditional herbs to help healing. We try to explain to the father that this type of practice won't help a fracture and encourage him to bring his children to the clinic first. We cleanse the wounds thoroughly, and we put the girl in a plaster of paris cast and encourage the father to bring his daughter back in the morning. I can only hope that the bones have been put back together well.

7:30 p.m.

I'm tired and ready to head back to the compound for dinner. As I do, gunshots begin filling the air just outside the compound. I worry that there might be fighting going on over the food that has been dropped by the World Food Program. We have had a large number of soldiers hanging around here this past week. We figure they heard about the food drop and have come to get some for themselves. The residents are powerless against them, and it stirs up quite a bit of anger. I also hope that it is nothing more serious because southern Sudan is in a precarious time of peace. We are all relieved when we learn that the shots were fired by two drunken soldiers. Even so, we hope that the peace will remain and that southern Sudan will finally begin to develop and prosper.

Catherine Hoelzer works with Christian Mission Aid in the upper Nile region of southern Sudan. She has indicated no relationships to disclose relating to the content of this piece.

Reprinted, with, from the *Journal of the American Academy of Physician Assistants,* December 2006.

A DAY IN THE LIFE: QUEENSLAND, AUSTRALIA, PA INTEGRATION

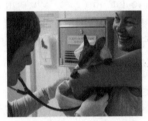

Nanette Laufik, PA-C

In September 2008, an ad appeared in the *Journal of the American Academy of Physician Assistants (JAAPA)*: "Exciting Opportunity for Physician Assistants in Queensland, Australia." Eight months later, I left for Cooktown, Australia, to participate in a 12-month trial that would introduce physician assistants (PAs) to Queensland.

A vast, largely rural, 668,000-square-mile state in northeast Australia, Queensland has a population of 4.3 million and is bordered by the 1,200-mile-long Great Barrier Reef. Many remote and rural communities in Queensland have difficulty attracting and retaining doctors. The PA concept was recognized as one possible solution to this chronic healthcare shortage. Cooktown, a small community of 1,500 located on the Coral Sea in far north Queensland, is 50 percent aboriginal. This small town also serves a "bush" area of another 1,500 people, including two indigenous communities and visiting tourists.

7:45 a.m.

Every morning I walk two-thirds of a mile to the Cooktown Multipurpose Health Centre. After nearly a year in the tropics, I remain disoriented by the reversed seasons. As the dry season of "winter" approaches, I notice the decrease in morning temperatures and humidity. Today will reach 27°C (80°F). It's Saturday, so traffic is light. Most drivers give a friendly wave. The recent increase in campervans means that the tourist season is *full on* (very busy). Gray nomads especially are escaping the colder south.

8:00 a.m.

The Friday night doctor-on-call reports the status of hospitalized patients and newly admitted patients to the weekend doctor and me. Our hospital has 14 acute beds and a 14-bed aged-care facility named Sunbird Cottage. Every other weekend I cover the outpatient department (OPD) and emergency department (ED) and help manage inpatients. There are no scheduled appointments on weekends, but I sometimes see recalls from earlier in the week. Working weekends is a win-win situation: We practice more autonomously, as we're accustomed to in the United States. The doctor-on-call spends more of her or his weekend at home, available by phone.

There have been two admissions so far this morning. The first is a middle-aged man with chronic pain issues, anxiety, and a history of drug addiction. He wants a head computed tomographic (CT) scan for an alleged injury sustained during an altercation that occurred 3 weeks ago. There have been no abnormal neurologic findings. If we refer him, the closest place for a CT scan is Cairns Base Hospital—a 3½-hour drive or 1-hour flight. The other admission is an 8-month-old with cough and fever brought in by his maternal grandmother. The threshold for admission is low here for babies, especially when there are complicating social issues.

8:20 a.m.

Inpatient rounds begin, and we see the 8-month-old baby first. He has just finished breakfast and has been wetting his *nappies* (diapers) frequently. He looks well and has no fever after two doses of paracetamol (acetaminophen). His mother has arrived, so the grandmother has gone home to rest. The mother is a tiny, quiet 18-year-old aboriginal who looks 13 and bewildered. She is pregnant again, and the young father is in trouble with the police. Grandmothers hold together many such tenuous families.

8:30 a.m.

A man in his late sixties who appears much older is next. He returned earlier this morning by commercial flight from Cairns, a city in Far North Queensland, where the Royal Flying Doctor Service (RFDS) had flown him 3 days ago for a chest CT scan. The RFDS—an Australian icon—provides free air ambulance service. Partly dependent on private donations, the service has been helping seriously ill and injured people in remote locations of Australia since 1928. Before this trip, our patient had presented with exacerbation of chronic obstructive pulmonary disease (COPD), pneumonia, a 90 pack-year smoking history, and an ominous-looking chest x-ray. The CT scan confirmed a diagnosis of lung cancer. He has opted for palliative care. Because he lives "out bush," he will stay here until transportation can be arranged. A shocking number of people here are heavy smokers. COPD and cancer are frustratingly common.

8:45 a.m.

Next, we see a 76-year-old man with late-onset schizophrenia. He is being managed with the help of a psychiatrist in Sydney, a 3-hour flight away. Since he lives alone and is located 45 minutes away, he will remain hospitalized during titration of his antipsychotic medications. He seems better and has not verbalized psychotic or paranoid thoughts for a few days, but I think he's in the "twilight zone" of therapeutic drug levels. I have a former psychiatric nurse gut feeling that he's guarding.

8:55 a.m.

A middle-aged aboriginal woman is here for abdominal pain, most likely caused by recurrent cholecystitis. She is overweight with poorly controlled diabetes, and this morning her fasting glucose level is 13.4 mmol/L (240 mg/dL). Adjusting insulin and other medications is a conundrum because patient compliance is often inconsistent. All patients have access to visiting specialist and diabetes teaching appointments that are free of charge.

10:20 a.m.

As I finish seeing patients and work on inpatient chart notes, my supervisor goes home. Next, a 41-year-old aboriginal stockman presents with exacerbation of asthma. He's an ex-smoker, but recently blooming wattle trees and smoke from a small bushfire have made him short of breath. While he receives the nebulized treatment I ordered for him, I am summoned back to the ward. An 85-year-old has just suffered a *transient ischemic* attack. He's had several attacks in the past 3 weeks, which necessitated his transfer here from Sunbird Cottage. We're all anticipating a fatal stroke. He is stable but drowsy. I return to the ED.

10:45 a.m.

Good improvement is seen in our asthmatic patient after one nebulized treatment. I supply him with oral prednisone and a replacement albuterol inhaler from our hospital pharmacy (sans pharmacist) and discharge him. On weekdays, I would have written a prescription to be signed by a doctor and filled by the local private pharmacist. Current laws for PA practice in Australia do not extend to federal pharmaceutical subsidies that patients receive for drugs. The law will change in time as PA practice evolves. For now, it's aggravating, but we deal with it.

12:30 p.m.

After lunch, I return to the OPD/ED. A tourist who had a heart valve replaced 6 months ago and is taking warfarin presents to have his international normalized ratio (INR) measured. This is another advantage of Australia's national health system: Patients can be seen at any hospital, free of charge, without appointments. The patient is grateful for his short wait time of 45 minutes. Another goal of introducing PAs in Queensland is to shorten waiting times in EDs, and this patient has experienced this benefit firsthand.

2:30 p.m.

In the past 2 hours I've seen a 4-year-old with otitis media, her 7-year-old brother with a mildly infected rash, and a 17-year-old with otitis externa, known here as "tropical ear." I also see a 5-year-old with a minor foot injury that does not require an x-ray. Considering how many children and adults regularly go barefooted here, the occurrence of foot injuries seems surprisingly low.

3:15 p.m.

A 32-year-old fisherman is brought in by one of his *mates* (friends) with a large, infected boil on his calf. Boils and cellulitis are extremely frequent among fisherman, and resistant Staphylococcus is frighteningly common and virulent. Shared showers, suboptimal immune systems (e.g., heavy smokers and binge drinkers), and sharing antibiotics while at sea all result in easy spread of disease and increased resistance to antibiotics.

4:25 p.m.

I'm nearly ready to leave for the day when a 34-year-old tourist presents with a marine sting on the top of his foot. He never saw the offending creature, but he poured a liter of vinegar, the recommended treatment for jellyfish stings, on his foot immediately.

The nurse and I pour another liter of vinegar on his foot and then apply an ice pack. The pain worsens. I ask the nurse to immerse his foot in hot water. The pain reduces. His response to the treatment leads to the correct diagnosis: He was stung by the barbed tail of a stingray, not a jellyfish. His tetanus immunization is current. He declines prophylactic antibiotics but will continue to soak his foot. Since he is staying with relatives locally and seems *clicked in* (aware and compliant), I trust that he'll return if signs of infection occur.

4:50 p.m.

I am pleased that I've learned enough tropical medicine to allow the doctor to enjoy her afternoon at home. I sign off by phone and wish her an uneventful night.

Nanette Laufik worked at Cooktown Multipurpose Health Centre in Queensland, Australia, at the time this article was written as part of a trial to introduce PAs to remote regions in the area. She is currently a senior lecturer/clinical skills coordinator at James Cook University School of Medicine in Cairns, Queensland, Australia. The author has indicated no relationships to disclose relating to the content of this article.

Reprinted, with permission, from the *Journal of the American Academy of Physician Assistants*, February 2010.

A DAY IN THE LIFE: ORTHOPEDICS IN LONDON, ENGLAND

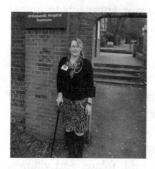

Kaatje van der Gaarden, PA-C

The Royal National Orthopaedic Hospital is located just outside London, England. When in November 2009, I came across an opportunity to work at its nationally acclaimed Spinal Cord Injury Centre, I immediately applied. Once known as "The Cure of Crippled Children Centre," the hospital is spread across buildings constructed in the 1920s. Americans also erected Nissen huts in the early 1940s. Made from corrugated steel, the prefabricated huts, which are similar to Quonset huts, are used as patient wards. The hospital is due for a much-needed renovation, starting next year.

8:15 a.m.

I live on site in the accommodations provided by the hospital, so my commute takes about 2 minutes. As always, I start the day with an American-size mug of Earl Grey tea with milk. I report directly to one of the consultants (supervising physicians), each of whom is responsible for half the 30 patients. I am lucky to work with Hajeena, an excellent junior doctor (resident). Although we share the same duties, I sometimes have additional responsibilities, such as the outpatient clinic and writing discharge reports. Patients are mainly spread out over two wards: rehabilitation in the Spinal Injury Unit (SIU) and prevention and care of bed sores in the Angus McKinnon Unit (AMU). Duties center around admitting a newly diagnosed *paraplegic* or *tetraplegic* patient, neurologic assessments, and managing a broad range of medical issues such as pneumonias and urinary tract infections (UTIs).

8:30 a.m.

Rebecca, the ward sister (senior nurse), and I discuss Mr. L outside his room. Mr. L is 60 years old and has tetraplegia, *ankylosing spondylitis*, schizophrenia, and *dysphagia*. He receives humidified oxygen through a *tracheotomy* because he is incapable of swallowing even saliva. Several neurologists, the speech-language therapist, gastroenterologist, and anesthesiologist have evaluated Mr. L without finding the etiology of the dysphagia. Computed tomographic (CT) scan and video swallowing studies show a lack of coordination and immobile pharyngeal muscles. One possibility is postoperative complications arising from an anterior approach to spinal fixation. Mr. L needs constant suctioning and has severe *hematuria*.

9:15 a.m.

I need to monitor Mr. L's *hemoglobin*. Nurses do not take blood samples or start intravenous (IV) lines on this ward, so after "bleeding" the patient, I fill out the requisition form and put the blood tubes in the attached plastic bag. The bag is then sent to the in-house pathology laboratory. Urine samples and nonroutine laboratory tests, such as thyroid, folate, and vitamin B_{12} determinations, are sent by taxis to a nearby hospital. Because the system is elaborate and samples do go missing, I call to ensure that the samples for blood cultures or other urgent requests have arrived. After documenting tests in Mr. L's paper medical record (there is no electronic record), I continue with the daily ward round.

9:45 a.m.

Ms. T has C5 tetraplegia after a truck hit her in a parking lot. She remembers her accident clearly and felt her neck break. Ms. T is in week 11 of her rehabilitation and has developed *neuropathic* pain, which arises in 80 percent of spinal-injury patients. Neuropathic pain is debilitating in itself, with only one-third of patients responding to medications. Ms. T and I decide to try her on pregabalin 75 mg at night. I write the medication on the chart and hand it over to the junior doctor or consultant, who cosigns. Physician assistants (PAs) do not have prescription rights in the United Kingdom. I find this difficult because the wards are very spread out, and some days I feel as if I am constantly hunting down my colleagues for signatures.

10:30 a.m.

After completing the documentation for patients at SIU, I'm off to AMU, the ward specializing in tissue viability, or pressure-sore management. Unfortunately, pressure sores in spinal-injury patients can take up to a year to heal. I take my down coat and brace myself for the cold because only makeshift hallways connect the wards. I go down the steep slope shivering and arrive at a warm AMU. Sunita, an experienced ward sister, requests a new drug chart for Mr. S. Every patient has a paper chart that has to be rewritten about once every month when it is full (which requires cosignatures). I also check on Mr. S, who has no new complaints. He was admitted with a grade 4 pressure sore and *osteomyelitis*. While in hospital, he spilled hot coffee over his right lower leg and required a skin graft for the burn. Both the donor site on his right thigh and the burn wound are healing quite nicely.

11:30 a.m.

I check the inpatient lab results. Mr. L's hemoglobin is 7.9 percent. The consultant, Dr. Gawronski, advises holding off on blood transfusion and repeating blood tests in 48 hours. I reply to internal e-mails and call a surgical specialty registrar. Most of our patients wear a body brace after neurosurgery, and the surgical team determines when the brace can be safely removed. I ask the specialty registrar to see Mr. P, who is anxious to have his cervicothoracolumbosacral body brace removed.

12:00 Noon

Tomorrow morning is the weekly consultant ward round, so I follow up on pending radiology and laboratory results. Dr. Gawronski, a nurse, and I will evaluate the progress of each patient, look at pressure sores, prescribe, and overall manage care. This ward round is followed by a multidisciplinary team meeting that includes the consultants, psychiatrist, social worker, nurse, psychologist, rehabilitation assistants, physiotherapists, and occupational therapists.

1:00 p.m.

I receive a beep regarding an admission for rehabilitation. Ms. C is a kind, elderly Indian woman who is recovering from spinal fixation for a lumbar fracture. The American Spinal Injury Association has developed an examination to determine the level of spinal injury. The examination is used worldwide as the most important diagnostic and prognostic indicator. Ms. C has an L5 incomplete spinal injury. I document the results of her physical examination and a cognitive screen and take a psychosocial history. Typically, a spinal-injury patient will arrive from other hospitals after stabilization, undergo neurosurgery and spine decompression here, and then go through a rehabilitation process that can take 8 weeks for incomplete paraplegia up to 6 months for complete tetraplegia. After teaching Ms. C about bladder and bowel management, including intermittent catheterization, I head back out in the cold and take another hallway to reach the outpatient clinic, where I spend the next part of my day.

2:00 p.m.

Once a week I see patients in the outpatient clinic. These patients have done their rehabilitation here and are seen for a yearly checkup. Because spinal-injury patients are at a higher risk of cardiovascular disease and *osteoporosis*, this may include ordering *dual-energy x-ray absorptiometry (DEXA)*, routine labs, and lipid determinations or providing health counseling. I review the two scheduled patients and check pending lab results.

3:30 p.m.

Mr. W comes in with his wife; both have paraplegia. Mr. W is 38 years old and has been bothered by abdominal pain for the past 6 months. The stomach pain exacerbates his *spasms* and neuropathic pain. He denies any first-degree family history of colon cancer, prior irritable bowel symptoms, rectal bleeding, change in bowel habits, fever, or weight loss. An abdominal examination detects normal bowel sounds and left lower quadrant tenderness. I fill out laboratory requests and once again regret that occult blood testing is not available in the hospital. On the recommendation of Dr. Gawronski, I order a CT scan and dictate a referral letter to the gastroenterologist. There is an online system for ordering and checking radiology results. Mr. W's blood will be drawn today, and I will follow up with a phone call or letter. I am beeped by the SIU that one of the patients has *pyrexia*. After checking with the consultant, I head to the ward immediately.

5:15 p.m.

I download the audio file and e-mail it to Dr. Gawronski's administrative assistant. She will transcribe the files the next day. Secretarial and administrative assistants are called PAs in the United Kingdom, and I hope this does not affect the implementation of physician assistants here. I bid Hajeena good night and head out. It's been another intense yet fulfilling day, and I look forward to swimming in the staff pool. Not a day goes by without my realizing that practicing in the United Kingdom is akin to the early days of our profession. It is a testimony to how much has been accomplished by PAs in the United States.

Kaatje van der Gaarden practiced rehabilitation medicine at the Spinal Cord Injury Centre, Royal National Orthopaedic Hospital, Stanmore, England, when this piece was written. She currently works for the gastro-enterology inpatient service at Presbyterian Hospital in Albuquerque, NM. Of note, she has an incomplete spinal cord injury. The author has indicated no relationships to disclose relating to the content of this piece.

Reprinted, with permission, from the *Journal of the American Academy of Physician Assistants*, December 2011.

A DAY IN THE LIFE: FAMILY PRACTICE IN THE UNITED KINGDOM

Lynn Tyrer, PA-C

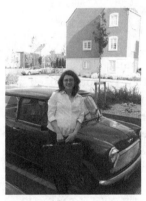

In September 2003, I started work as a physician assistant (PA) at a family-practice clinic in the United Kingdom. This clinic—or general-practice surgery, as it is called—is located in a low-income, high-need area, and the business partners had struggled to find a full-time physician to replace the one who had retired. Eventually, they turned to U.S.-trained PAs for a solution. On a smaller scale, their situation was not unlike the one that launched the PA profession in the United States, and they sought out a profession that has long been committed to providing care in underserved areas.

This was an exciting opportunity for me because I would be able to promote the profession on an international level. Since becoming a PA, I have passionately believed that we can help to meet medical needs worldwide—and I even found evidence supporting this belief when I wrote my research thesis as a student. I do believe that PAs will eventually have international representation and unification similar to other medical professions. I also wanted to practice in a country with a national health system so that

I could experience firsthand the pros and cons of such a system. And I wanted to be able to travel.

I was hired on a 2-year work contract. As part of the contract, I am also part of a pilot research project commissioned by the Changing Workforce Programme of the U.K. Department of Health. My days include working in the clinic, doing home visits (a routine part of the primary-care service here), attending meetings to assist in the promotion of the PA profession in the United Kingdom, and collecting and recording data as needed for the pilot study. I work on a team with two doctors, one nurse practitioner (who mainly sees patients with diabetes, chronic obstructive pulmonary disease, and asthma), and a practice nurse who performs duties similar to that of a licensed practical nurse (LPN). Nursing titles and nursing training differs from those in the United States.

9:00 a.m.

I arrive at the clinic and finish any paperwork not completed from the previous day. This time is also reserved for answering any incoming phone queries from patients.

9:30 a.m.

Clinic starts. I typically see 15 patients in the morning. The appointment times are set 10 minutes apart, with approximately 12 slots booked and 3 left open for patients requesting appointments that day. One of the new mandates set out by the U.K. National Health Service (NHS) is the access target. These targets were established in response to patient demand. For primary care, the mandate stipulates that a patient should be offered an appointment with a healthcare practitioner within 24 hours and an appointment with the doctor within 48 hours.

In addition, we have the new General Medical Service (GMS) II targets. These reflect clinical and administrative goals and reward good clinical practice. For example, points are given if 80 percent of diabetic patients on the practice register have an A1C level of less than 7.4 percent and if smoking status has been ascertained and cessation advice given for persons older than 16 years.

All goals set by the NHS ultimately are linked to reimbursement. Clinicians are encouraged to try to address the GMS II goals opportunistically when seeing patients. This is often difficult to manage in a 10-minute appointment with a patient who has two or more problems; however, so the practice makes the effort to schedule appointments specifically to address GMS II goals.

The range of patients and presenting problems that I see is similar to that of a PA working in the United States with a few exceptions. These include people requesting over-the-counter (OTC) medications (certain people qualify for free medicine) and those requesting "sick notes" (forms issued by the doctor signing a patient off of work). Sick notes are issued for varied reasons, but they can be given for conditions as simple as the common cold. Patients who are off work for more than 7 days need a note from their doctor explaining why.

Another difference in the NHS is data recording. Healthcare is moving toward a "paper-light" system, in which all information will be electronic and accessible via a national database. All patient information at our clinic, from administrative information to telephone conversations, is entered onto the computer. This includes all clinic appointments as well.

In the United States, the clinician typically knows why the patient is coming in; also, a nurse usually obtains needed equipment in advance and prepares the patient. In the U.K. system, however, a nurse does not see the patient first. Clinicians collect their own patient data (e.g., vital signs, weight, and peak flows) and also must prepare patients for examination and arrange for any necessary equipment. This process does affect the schedule, and patients sometimes must book new appointments for further data collection and management.

This morning in clinic, the presenting problems I saw were *hyperemesis* in pregnancy (I referred the patient to secondary care for inpatient treatment), a few coughs and sore throats, increased shortness of breath in a patient with chronic obstructive pulmonary disease (COPD) and congestive heart failure (CHF), low back pain (two patients), *menorrhagia*, a *Pap smear* and well-woman check, blood pressure (BP) management, breast lump, rectal bleeding, depression (two patients), and a few rashes.

12:30 to 3:30 p.m.

This time is reserved for administrative work but is usually an extension of clinical tasks. Initially, I complete any referrals to specialists or consultants that arose from the morning clinic. Then I go through laboratory and radiology results, both of which are again recorded on the computer. Following this, I respond to patient telephone inquiries and medication requests that reception staff recorded that morning, as well as question or approve any medication changes recommended in secondary care. If any home-visit requests have come in for the morning, these are divided between the doctor and me. On average, we usually have about three requests a day. Much of the 3 hours between morning and afternoon clinic can be taken up with home visits. I try to take 30 minutes for lunch—and if there is time left over, I spend it doing administrative tasks such as medication reviews.

3:30 to 6:00 p.m.

This is evening clinic, where again I am booked for 10-minute appointments. Generally, I have 11 appointments during evening clinic—most prebooked. I saw a similar range of patients this afternoon as I did this morning with a few exceptions. One patient was specifically booked for a medication review (which helped to capture information for the GMS II targets), and one was booked for a double appointment to fill out an insurance claim form. Following my last patient, I complete any consultant referrals, review laboratory results, and respond to any patient inquiries.

Frustrations and Rewards

I have encountered some frustrations practicing as a PA in the United Kingdom. Primarily, these include the waiting lists and the growing pains associated with starting up an old profession in a new country.

Patients sometimes must wait for 6 months or more before they can see a specialist. The waiting lists for some radiology studies, such as ultrasonography, are also up to 6 months. More detailed imaging studies, such as CT scans and magnetic resonance imaging (MRI), can be ordered only by specialists; even primary-care physicians are not permitted to order these tests. On a professional level, the local radiology department has not approved PAs working in primary care to order radiographs, so we must obtain a signature from our supervising doctor. The same goes for prescribing medications. Despite these frustrations, the rewards have been worth the sacrifices.

About 18 U.S.-trained PAs are currently working here in the United Kingdom, with a further 11 to start soon. Most are working in primary care, and some are working secondary care in emergency settings. Each PA may be used in different ways depending on clinic setting and team decisions.

My experience has been educational, rewarding, and challenging, and I am proud to have worked with other PAs, as well as with forward-thinking U.K. clinicians, to promote the PA profession "across the pond."

Lynn Tyrer works as a PA in Tipton, England, which is near Birmingham. She has indicated no relationships to disclose relating to the content of this piece.

Reprinted, with permission, from the *Journal of the American Academy of Physician Assistants,* August 2005.

TEACHING AND RESEARCH

A DAY IN THE LIFE: PA PROFESSOR AND ORTHOPEDIC CLINICIAN

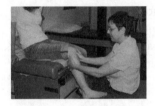

Dawn Colomb-Lippa, PA-C

Many years ago, when I was planning a career change, I knew one thing for sure: I wanted to teach. I knew that my next move had to put me in a field in which education was guided by practitioners. I wanted to be able to help students learn what seemed unlearnable—and for me, that was teaching gross anatomy. Now I spend my days playing multiple roles: physician assistant (PA) professor, orthopedic clinician, and mother. There is really no such thing as an "average" day in my world, but here I try to describe as close to my average day as I can.

6:45 a.m.

Today is the first day of lab, and I should be on my way, but I forgot my notes, as usual, and so I have stopped off at the PA program. A full hour before lab is supposed to begin, a small group of unfamiliar faces is gathering here in Hamden—but the lab is downtown in New Haven. I guess they are carpooling. These students, although unknown to me now, within 2 weeks' time will be as familiar to me as my own children. We are about to begin a semester of human anatomy together, which will bind us in a shared experience forever. My role as an academic advisor begins early this year because one of the students on my list seems anxious. "Can I talk to you for a minute, Professor Colomb-Lippa?" He doesn't know yet to call me what everyone does—Professor CL. After some sputtering, he confides that he is nervous about dissecting an actual human. His grandfather just died this spring, and he thinks the dissection might be difficult for him. I advise him to keep his mind on the science of the dissection and to try to remember how supportive his grandfather would be of him as he begins his training as a PA. And, as an afterthought, I ask him to let me know if he is going to pass out. He seems to feel a bit better, but we'll see.

7:15 a.m.

I park in a municipal parking lot and begin the quarter-mile hike to the lab. My backpack is filled with a portable autopsy saw, scalpels, a change of clothing, and a human skull. I hope to high heaven that I don't get frisked by one of the New Haven bicycle cops. When I get to the lab, I am greeted by the mortician, a man I have known for 11 years now. He tells me that there is a crowd of nervous-looking young adults forming outside the lab. Without having met them before, it is clear to me that they are my new PA class. Bright faces, eager to learn, with a slight hint of fear. "Good," I think. "They are ready to begin."

7:30 a.m.

I have changed, and I enter the lab. Not one of the now over 50 students in the hallway follows me. Entering the lab alone, the quiet feels almost holy. It may seem strange, but this feels like home to me. I open the lab table and begin the process of unsheathing the cadaver. The students' faces pop into view through the small window in the door. I signal for them to come in. Slowly, they filter in, some in scrubs, some in T-shirts with obscure sayings on them. I am getting old, no doubt. The students register that I am now standing in front of a prosected dead human. I assign them to tables in groups, and the realization of the fact that they, too, will be dissecting a human is evident on their faces. I spew the opening phrases of lab, including the rules and regulations, the need for respect of the body, and an overview of the tremendous task we are about to begin. My lab instructors help the students open the tables and meet the gift that has been left to them by people they will never meet.

2:00 p.m.

The entire class survived the first cadaver lab unscathed, including my advisee who lost his grandpa just before arriving at PA school. The students have completed the full posterior dissection of muscles and spinal cord, and now they change their clothing and leave for another class on campus. I feel bad for their electrocardiogram (ECG) professor because I know the class is tired, and they smell. A student stops to ask me if she can make an appointment to meet just to be sure she gets off to a good start in her summer classes. She quietly confesses that she has a learning disability and doesn't want to fall behind. We set a day and time to meet. This is a proactive student, I think to myself, but she has a long haul ahead of her. I will refer her to the Learning Center, among other things.

I clean up, make a quick phone call to the PA program to be sure that no students have withdrawn after today's muscle and bone marathon, and change my clothes in order to head to my clinical job as an orthopedic PA.

3:00 p.m.

Generally, I am nearing the end of my 9-hour clinical day by now, but today I am coming in to see a few quick patients who were scheduled to see one of my supervising physicians. A trauma threw off the operating room (OR) schedule, and Dr. F is just beginning the *arthroscopy* that was scheduled for 10:00 a.m. I start with Mrs. M, an older woman who is known to the practice for years now. Her *degenerative joint disease* has worsened in her right knee. It's time for a replacement, but like so many folks in her situation, she is 100 pounds overweight and pushing a deadline: Her son is getting married in 2 months, and she would like to be mobile for the event. I give her a steroid injection and set her up to come back in 2 weeks to talk surgery with the doctor. I know the steroid will do little good, but it will give her time (and evidence) to decide on a replacement sooner rather than later.

3:15 p.m.

Two quick viscosupplementation injections and on to Mr. F, a 14-year-old runner with hip pain. I am meeting him for the first time today, but it is clear to me that his mother is worried about his complaint and equally clear that he is not going to stop running anytime soon. His exam shows some joint *laxity*, asymmetry of hip alignment, and a thoracic *scoliosis*. When I mention the "s word," his mother becomes even more concerned. The patient's sister had terrible scoliosis requiring surgical correction, and Mr. F just "passed" a scoliosis screening at school this week. I send him off for some x-rays. I'll call the mother tomorrow with the results, which no doubt will be positive.

3:45 p.m.

A phone call: Ms. C just had a mini–open rotator cuff repair, and she wants to know if she can take off her sling. Also, she has questions about "what exactly was done" in the OR. This will not be a quick one. I convince her that she needs to wear that unfriendly sling for another 4 or 5 weeks, and I give my best simplified explanation of the functional anatomy of the rotator cuff (a subject covered in several hours of lab and lecture for my PA students), followed by a crash course in the use of biodegradable anchors in cuff repair (a subject covered in years of orthopedic fellowship). She buys it. I will see her next week to get her stitches out and start her in physical therapy (PT).

4:00 p.m.

An add-in: Mr. R, a patient of ours, has fractured his foot at work and was seen several days ago in the emergency department. He brings his films with him, which show a Jones fracture of his left foot. He has never been told he has diabetes, but he also does not see a primary-care provider. He says that he has "circulation issues," which spells "undiagnosed diabetes" or "peripheral vascular disease" to me, either one a bad indicator of this fracture's ability to heal with conservative treatment. I talk to him about the options and the possibility of failure of conservative treatment. Nonetheless, he does not want to have an operation if not needed. I put him in a non-weight-bearing short-leg cast as a trial and give him crutches. I'll see him in 3 weeks and see what's going on at that fracture sight. My fingers are crossed!

4:15 p.m.

Mr. R was my last patient of the day, so I have a quick look around to see the mess of charts and equipment I need to straighten up. "Leave it; I'll get it," I hear. Thank goodness for our wonderful medical assistants because I do have to shoot out and get my 4-year-old from day care and meet my 6-year-old at the bus stop. Now I begin my third job: mother. This one pays very little, but the benefits are amazing. And I think there may be room for advancement someday (grandmother!).

7:30 p.m.

I put my daughters to sleep and quickly check my e-mails—which often is a mistake. I have 24 new messages since 2 p.m., and many of them are from students. Most have questions. Which atlas is best for comparing structures? What is the website for ordering those thick gloves? One catches my eye. In the subject line, it says, "Thanks." It's from my advisee. He wanted to thank me for meeting with him this morning. He was nervous, but he did fine in lab and is really excited to go to open lab tomorrow night to review structures. He also says that I was right—his grandfather would be proud of him—and he thanks me again. I am glad I checked my e-mails.

Dawn Colomb-Lippa is Professor of Physician Assistant Studies at Quinnipiac University, Hamden, CT, practices orthopedics at Tribury Orthopaedics, Waterbury, CT, and is a member of the Journal of the American Academy of Physician Assistants editorial board.

Reprinted, with permission, from the *Journal of the American Academy of Physician Assistants*, June 2008.

A DAY IN THE LIFE: CLINICAL PRACTICE AND RESEARCH IN NEUROLOGY

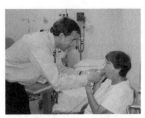

James M. Taft, PA-C

When I was in physician assistant (PA) school at SUNY Stonybrook, I always thought I would practice emergency medicine or family medicine after I graduated. I never envisioned the combination of clinical practice and research in neurology that currently fills my days. In 1984 (now I really date myself), there were few jobs for PAs in emergency medicine, so I took a job in neuromuscular research at the New England Medical Center in Boston. After a few years, I managed to find a position in emergency medicine, where I stayed for over 10 years. Then the emergency room (ER) started to change, and all the PAs headed to the new fast track. I knew I wouldn't be happy doing that too, so I went back to neurology.

My site collaborates with Massachusetts General Hospital in Boston on a number of different research studies in patients with *amyotrophic lateral* sclerosis (ALS). As part of the project team, I troubleshoot the pulmonary function machines and oversee other outcome measurements for all 27 study sites nationwide. My clinical duties include ALS clinic, headache clinic, and general neurology. My time is divided equally between research and clinical medicine. Here is a day in the life of a clinical and research PA.

7:30 a.m.

I arrive at my office and sift through my e-mails and voice mails. This morning, there are a few from study sites having problems with their pulmonary function machines. There are also a number of e-mails from patients in regard to medication refills and problems or questions they have. This has become a popular method of communication for my patients and is especially convenient for those with ALS because most of them cannot talk. The easy exchange of information via e-mail has enhanced patient care. After I answer each patient's message, I print off a copy to go into the clinical record.

8:00 a.m.

We currently have four research studies ongoing. Today I'm seeing three ALS patients who are enrolled in clinical trials. All the trials are double-blind and placebo-controlled, which can be tough on the patients. These studies focus on slowing disease progression, which is why outcome measures are so important. We do not have a clear enough understanding of the pathophysiology of the disease to look for a cure, but hopefully we will soon. Each study has a unique protocol, with scheduled visits for vital sign and *vital capacity* measurements, blood and urine collections, electrocardiograms (ECGs), and quality-of-life measurement. Each visit also includes physical and neurologic exams, which take 1 to 2 hours per patient. Even though these are research visits, I go over clinical issues too, including medications and physical therapy equipment such as walkers or wheelchairs.

Study visits with ALS patients usually require attending to their social needs as well as to their physical condition. One patient I see has a vital capacity of 20 percent even on bilevel positive airway pressure (BIPAP). We talk about death and dying, and I go over all the options, from life support to hospice care. The patient and family choose hospice, and I will call them later to make the referral. I give them a script for lorazepam and will mail one for liquid morphine. Air hunger can be very distressing, and these drugs can ease symptoms and make the patient more comfortable. I have been caring for this patient for 3 years now, and I know him and his family well. I experience the emotional rollercoaster of their situation along with them.

My patients with ALS are dying, and I do my best to get in some laughs and goofy jokes during their research visits. I have a weird sense of humor—patients and families often tell me that it helps them through this dark time. All my ALS patients get hugs. Even the men. Even during difficult conversations, patients and families can be crying one minute and laughing the next.

I occasionally make house calls to see patients with ALS. I find house calls interesting because the families invite me into their home and treat me like one of the family. The visits usually take about an hour but can last much longer if I let them. Patients and families love it when I make a house call, and they shower me with food—especially cookies. I never refuse, of course! We talk about current problems and issues, and I examine the patient. I try to have the hospice nurse at the visit to make sure that all of us are on the same page.

Recently, I saw an ALS patient at home who was having difficulty swallowing but who had decided against a feeding tube. The hospice nurse had advised her not to eat potato chips, but this was the patient's favorite food. I took out my pad and wrote a prescription for her to have one bag of potato chips per day. This was a big hit with the family and is now a standing joke with the hospice nurses. Sometimes it's the little things that make the patients' and families' difficult times a little easier.

11:30 a.m.

The research patient visits are complete, but I have a few hours' worth of paperwork and data entry to complete. Most studies are web-based, so after filling out the clinical research forms, I enter the data on the study's website. As I do this, I multitask, simultaneously making a few phone calls or answering e-mails.

12:10 p.m.

I eat a quick lunch at my desk as I review the latest headline news updates. I sometimes search for articles on patient safety for the American Academy of Physician Assistants (AAPA) Quality Care Committee, of which I am a member.

12:45 p.m.

I leave for the headache clinic, located a 10-minute walk from my office across the busiest intersection in Syracuse. The clinic is made up of one physician and me, and we usually see 18 to 24 patients in 4 hours. We are the only tertiary-care headache clinic in seven counties. A quick schedule check reveals 16 follow-up patients—not too bad. Most have primary headache syndromes, including migraine with and without *aura*, chronic daily headache, or analgesic rebound. I try to put patients on preventive medications, empower them to control their headaches through lifestyle changes, and limit their use of over-the-counter (OTC) drugs.

   At the headache clinic, I move from room to room, visiting the familiar faces. I see a 56-year-old man who had chronic daily headaches for 6 years without relief. His new preventive medication has given him periods of no headaches for up to 10 days. But not all the cases are that easy. There are a few I am still having trouble controlling, despite trying multiple medications. Some patients have only periodic headaches and just need medication refills. Others seem to come in only to catch up on the gossip. All get a brief neurologic exam. I find myself discussing herbal alternatives, and I tell them which have been shown to be effective and which are ineffective or dangerous. Finally, I review diet journals at each visit, check caffeine use, and assess use of OTC medications with an eye for analgesic rebound.

4:30 p.m.

I've seen my last patient, and now I find myself staring at a pile of charts to dictate. Unfortunately, there is no time between patients to get the dictations done, so I pick up the phone and get started.

5:00 p.m.

I'm back in my office doing one final sort through the e-mails and voice mails. I answer the ones that can't wait until the morning. An hour or two of research data sits on my desk, waiting to be entered online. But, for now, I'm tired, and the data isn't going anywhere.

As I head home, I often think about the day. For example, did I forget to do something? What else can I do for a patient's headache when most treatments have failed? Occasionally, I have a brainstorm and call the patient the next day. But most of the time I reflect on the ALS patients and their constant struggle, every day, not only fighting the disease but also fighting with insurance companies and the government to get the most basic kind of help, such as wheelchairs. Patients with ALS face difficult times, yet they smile, laugh, and thank me for my time. It sounds corny, but I'm happy just to be a part of their lives.

James M. Taft practices at SUNY Upstate Medical University, Syracuse, NY. He has indicated no relationships to disclose relating to the content of this piece.

Reprinted, with permission, from the *Journal of the American Academy of Physician Assistants*, October 2006.

A DAY IN THE LIFE: CLINICAL AND HEALTH RESEARCH

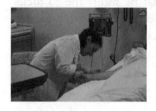

Alexandra Braunstein Scott, MS, PA-C, MPH

I work in the Michigan Clinical Research Unit (MCRU), a human clinical trial unit at the University of Michigan Hospital. MCRU provides the resources and infrastructure needed to conduct clinical research protocols and is sponsored by the Michigan Institute for Clinical and Health Research (MICHR). MICHR provides a wide variety of programs and services for University of Michigan investigators who are conducting clinical or translational research. Our research volunteers include both healthy persons as well as people with diseases refractory to standard treatments. Unlike the rest of the hospital, most of our patients are not acutely ill.

8:00 a.m.

I look over today's schedule, which is particularly busy. A good portion of my time involves performing history and physical exams (H&Ps) of study participants as part of the study screenings. I see that several participants will be receiving an infusion today. Although I am not involved directly with most infusions, I read the medical histories of the participants and familiarize myself with the type of infusion they will receive. One of the goals of these studies is to determine safety and tolerability of the agent; therefore, we need to be prepared to treat allergic reactions. Some of the participants will receive a placebo, but I won't know who they are because this is a double-blind study. I also read about the studies to remind myself of the goals, purposes, and interventions of the various protocols in order to tailor my exams appropriately. Mary, my nurse practitioner (NP) counterpart, and I divide the schedule up between us.

9:00 a.m.

I attend an initiation meeting to discuss an upcoming study with the principal investigator (PI) and study coordinators. Some members of our research unit—including a nurse manager, a clinical nurse specialist, a lead lab technician, a bionutritionist, a pharmacist, an administrative assistant, an NP, and a PA—attend these meetings. We discuss the requirements for nursing assistance, lab draws, physical exams, diets, specimen processing, scheduling, and billing with the study team. This particular study protocol is on depression and associated emotional processing and neurotransmitter functioning. The PI tells me that he wants me to focus on any medical reasons for depression that the participants may have when I examine them. For comparison, I also will be examining nondepressed control subjects.

9:45 a.m.

A 32-year-old woman with metastatic *sarcoma* has arrived for her experimental treatment with Reolysin, a reovirus being tested in cancer patients. This is her second day of the 5-day treatment regimen. I briefly assess her for side effects. She tells me that overnight she had a headache and low-grade fever but is feeling better this morning. (Flulike symptoms are a common side effect of Reolysin.) I also check her lab results and call her oncologist to ensure that she is stable enough to receive another dose of the drug today. Many of us at the research center know this young woman, a mother of three, because she has been coming here for monthly treatments. We all pray that this regimen will finally prove effective for her.

10:00 a.m.

My first H&P of the day is for an overweight 12-year-old girl. She is participating in a study on screening for prediabetes and diabetes in children and adolescents. The nurses have already inserted an intravenous (IV) line and started an oral glucose tolerance test. Today she also will receive dietary counseling from one of our bionutritionists. I carefully examine her skin folds for *acanthosis* nigricans, the darkened skin pigmentation associated with obesity and insulin resistance. As I examine her, I am reminded of the growing problem of obesity in children in our country. I hope that taking part in this study will help this child and her parents better understand the health risks of being overweight and be motivated to eat healthier and exercise.

10:45 a.m.

My next case requires a skin biopsy. This is a study on *scleroderma* and examines the inflammation and *fibrosis* of tissues caused by this disfiguring disease. The study participant is a middle-aged man with obvious hardened, thickened skin on his arms and face. The disease has affected his lungs as well. I look for a scleroderma-involved portion of his arm that is suitable for biopsy. After prepping an appropriate area of skin, I carefully inject lidocaine to numb the area. This is tricky because of the unyielding skin. I have to push the syringe harder than normal, and the lidocaine does not make its usual wheal that signals that the solution is in the skin. I proceed carefully with the punch biopsy to be sure that he is adequately anesthetized. His wife has agreed to be a control subject; therefore, my next task is to perform a skin biopsy on her.

12:00 Noon

I check in on one research subject who was admitted to our center for a 2-week stay. This is a normal, healthy graduate student who is taking part in a study of the relationship between growth hormone and weight regulation. Participants in this study are required to consume a high-calorie diet with limited activity for 2 weeks. This particular participant is feeling well physically but does appear quite bored after 5 days of this regimen. At the end of the study, she will undergo a muscle biopsy. Because I am learning how to perform this procedure, I will perform it with the study physician.

12:15 p.m.

I take a break to eat lunch, catch up on writing notes, and prepare for my afternoon appointments. My husband calls me to say hello and to ask if I petted the cat goodbye before leaving the house this morning.

1:15 p.m.

I perform a follow-up exam on a participant in a study that will determine the effectiveness of a low-salt diet on chronic kidney disease. With the guidance of the research dieticians, this 66-year-old man has been following a low-salt diet for the past month. During my exam, I focus on volume-status markers, including lower extremity edema, lung *crackles*, and jugular venous distension. Since I last saw him, his leg swelling has improved markedly, his blood pressure has improved, and he is feeling better. Bioelectrical impedance testing (done by the study team) confirms the improvements.

1:45 p.m.

My next participant has type 2 diabetes and is presenting for a screening visit for a study on peripheral *neuropathy*. I am careful to ask about the signs and symptoms of neuropathy and to assess neurologic functioning, including a monofilament foot exam. These study participants will also undergo further neuropathic testing in the hospital neurology lab.

2:30 p.m.

My last H&P of the day is for an alternative-medicine study involving the use of chamomile extract for chronic insomnia. I evaluate these study participants for secondary causes of insomnia, such as chronic pain and depression. Unfortunately, this study participant was a no-show. I joke with the staff that perhaps he was too tired to come today. In reality, however, there are many cancellations in the world of research. Our study participants are volunteers; many of them are generally healthy and often simply do not show up. Other participants present for their appointments but do not meet the inclusion criteria for the study. Some have decided not to participate after talking to the study team and reading the consent form. I take advantage of the extra time to do some medical reading.

3:30 p.m.

I communicate via e-mail to study teams to clarify their needs for upcoming studies. I assist the nursing staff with blood draws because a number of participants need labs at this particular time. I sign orders for a study participant arriving later this evening for an overnight admission. I also briefly review the next day's schedule. My first case for tomorrow is a *fistula* exam in a participant receiving an experimental treatment for *Crohn's disease*. In the afternoon I will be traveling to an offsite clinic to examine subjects with *fibromyalgia*.

4:30 p.m.

On the way home I reflect on how different my current position is from my frenetic years in inpatient internal medicine. I saw much suffering inside the hospital walls during that time. It is intriguing to think that I am now involved in studies that aim to develop new understandings and treatments for various medical conditions. Although it may take many more study subjects before results are known and several years before others can benefit, anticipation of what the outcomes might promise is exciting. I feel privileged to play a small role in these endeavors.

Alexandra Scott works in the Michigan Clinical Research Unit, University of Michigan Hospital, Ann Arbor, MI. The author has indicated no relationships to disclose relating to the content of this piece.

Reprinted, with permission, from the *Journal of the American Academy of Physician Assistants,* February 2010.

MILITARY

A DAY IN THE LIFE: AEROMEDICAL PA WITH THE ARMY NATIONAL COAST GUARD

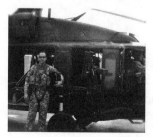

Major Shawn T. Buller, APA-C, MPH

The U.S. Army has recognized the importance of meeting the healthcare needs of aviators, who must maintain a high standard of physical fitness, since creation of the Army Air Corps before World War II. The *flight surgeon* is a clinician whose primary responsibility is the healthcare of personnel on flight status. An aeromedical physician assistant (APA-C) is a clinician who can fill the role of flight surgeon.

The training program for flight surgeons is designed to develop the clinician's ability to recognize potential medical problems or the sudden incapacitation of an aviator. Flight surgeons also fly a minimum number of hours in order to understand the effects of fatigue, vibration, and noise on an aviator. This is my second tour to Iraq but my first tour "on flight status."

10:00 p.m.

I am just back from flying a mission north of Baghdad. I am barely able to stand, and a wave of fatigue and nausea comes over me as I leave the Blackhawk helicopter. I am close to being a heat casualty after flying over the combat zone for 6 hours in 130-degree heat. I sit down on the edge of the runway and recall the events of the day, thankful to be back in familiar surroundings.

I remember one small forward operating base (FOB) we landed at for a short stay; the FOB was located along the border of Iran. Like every other combat outpost, it was blanketed with dust and surrounded by 15-foot-high cement walls.

I learned that the medics at this FOB were available only for sick call and emergent-care issues. I walked around in an attempt to link up with the medics. A sergeant at the base heard I was there and asked me to help the medics evaluate incoming injured coalition troops who had been involved in a motor vehicle rollover. I was directed to the medic tent and waited for the patients. I quickly triaged the patients' injuries, and the medics got to work treating their wounds, which appeared to be non-life-threatening orthopedic injuries. Nonetheless, the patients were stabilized and packaged up for medevac. I waited for the medevac helicopters to circle above and handed the situation over to the FOB medics because my crew was waiting for me. I could see the patients being loaded onto the medevac helicopters as we lifted off and circled above the base. Watching the scene below, I smiled to myself, knowing that I had really made a difference today.

8:00 a.m.

Back at my base in southern Iraq, I've dragged myself out of my bunk, and now I'm evaluating routine sick-call patients. Sick call includes almost everything you would see in the United States, conditions as mundane as athlete's foot to a sprained ankle. I give the medics some quick on-the-go tips on everything from pathophysiology to pharmacology while evaluating patients, which works out great because the patients appreciate the education as well.

11:30 a.m.

Before going to lunch, I double-check the list of soldiers given influenza immunizations. On arrival in Iraq, many soldiers were quarantined with flulike symptoms and subsequently tested positive for the flu. The remaining asymptomatic soldiers didn't want to get sick or be stuck in quarantine, so they all got their shots.

1:00 p.m.

When I return from the chow hall, I check the afternoon patient schedule; only two patients require a flight surgeon. One is an unmanned aerial vehicle (UAV) operator/pilot, and the other is a crew chief. The UAV pilot is an easy flight physical; he is healthy, and the evaluation is quick. Although pressed for time, I like to find out information, so I ask, "Anything interesting out there to see?" All the UAV pilots give the same answer: "No." I know they have to be pretty tight-lipped because of operational security, so I don't press the issue.

The crew chief presents for a recheck of what at first appeared to be some ulnar nerve symptoms. I had initially inquired about his positioning in the Blackhawk, which included sitting at the side of the helicopter holding onto a machine gun while leaning on his elbows out a side window. He was advised to use elbow pads and attempt a different position, one that does not involve leaning on his elbows; now he is returning to let me know that this seemed to help, and his symptoms are improved.

The medic reminds me that I am scheduled to work the emergency room (ER) by myself, which supports a base with more than 7,000 soldiers, sailors, marines, and airmen. The ER is supported by an on-call forward surgical team (FST) capable of handling most trauma patients who come through the door. Little did I know that this would be a night I would call for their help.

3:00 p.m.

I examine a group of soldiers who are ready to redeploy back to their home station. They have been in Iraq anywhere from 10 to 12 months and are here for a mandatory postdeployment health assessment (PDHA), which requires a face-to-face encounter with a clinician. The PDHA is designed to screen soldiers for disease, illness, or injuries that may have occurred during their deployment.

This group, Desert XI, is a military transition team that helps to train the local Iraqi and Afghan populations. The teams are typically made up of 10 to 14 soldiers from different job specialties and locations who are trained to be advisors. This particular group was based at the infamous Chemical Ali's house. Their common complaint is that the chemical fumes from the basement were so strong that no one could enter the area. Months earlier, a mass grave had been discovered in the front yard. The soldiers wanted to document that they had been exposed to fumes from burning trash and oil refineries or possibly chemical weapons that might pose long-term adverse health effects.

The consistently humid air in southern Iraq creates a thick early morning fog of burning trash fumes and the smell of oil refineries that burns your eyes and nostrils. Some soldiers present with asthma-like symptoms after trying to exercise. It makes me think about how awful it must be to grow up in this kind of pollution and what the long-term effects of exposure to these toxic fumes will be for us.

5:00 p.m.

After sending up reports and sitting through the unit's battle-update briefing, a biweekly meeting that helps the commanders and staff catch up on the latest changes, I find myself once again dreading my impending shift in the ER. I make my way to the dining facility and eventually back to my hooch to get ready for my long night.

8:00 p.m.

The night starts out quietly. The medics are meeting for the first time. Some have just arrived from the United States and have been in country for less than a week, and others were brought in from all over Iraq to help beef up the base's medical capabilities. Most are new graduates of medic school and have never been deployed to the combat zone.

4:00 a.m.

It's Sunday morning, and I am nearing the end of my shift. I have used the precious time to catch up on some paperwork. Suddenly, radio chatter begins: "Roger. We are in flight to your location." The ER phone rings, and a medic relays the call, "Sir, we have two casualties. One is urgent surgical and one is priority . . . both gunshot wounds." At once, everyone is alert and looking at me. I sit up and tell the medic, "Call the surgical team, lab, and x-ray. Now! One of you stay next to the radio; the rest come with me."

The medics follow me into the trauma room, which is a tent across from the ER. Our "hospital" is a bunch of tents hooked together. I start assigning the medics to different tasks. "I want everyone to put on a trauma gown and gloves." All the medics are very quiet, intent on not looking like they just graduated from medic school. They are wide-eyed, and their faces look expressionless, but they move with anticipation; each movement is deliberate, as if they are on the edge of panic. I then point to different medics: "I want you to check the monitors. You get the fluids ready. Get this place cleared and ready to accept patients."

At that point, the overworked FST starts to filter in; surgeons, nurses, x-ray, and lab personnel all quietly get their equipment prepared for the incoming patients. The patients, having arrived by helicopter, are soon transferred to the care of the trauma team. Everyone works diligently to stabilize the patients. I step aside and head back to the ER clinic, which is much quieter, and watch from a distance while the others work on the patients.

8:00 a.m.

My relief has arrived, and I put on my protective vest and helmet, grab my pistol, and head for the door. The fatigue sets in again as the adrenaline wears off. Another day gone by brings me another day closer to home.

Shawn Buller is an aeromedical physician assistant with the Army National Guard and was deployed to Iraq at the time this piece was written. When not on active duty, he practices emergency medicine in Charlotte, NC. He has indicated no relationships to disclose relating to the content of this piece.

Reprinted, with permission, from the *Journal of the American Academy of Physician Assistants,* April 2010.

CIVILIAN TACTICAL MEDICINE

Jefferey G. Yates, MPA, PA-C

Providing Emergent Care in Austere Environments

An interesting concept of delivering medical care—civilian tactical medicine—began to develop across the nation in the 1980s to deal with high-risk or potentially dangerous situations. Civilian tactical medicine first adopted the style of the military corpsman. Over the past 30 years, this concept has fully embraced the advancing methodology of military medicine along with the philosophy of civilian prehospital care. As the tactical medic team leader of the Portsmouth Police Department SWAT team in Portsmouth, VA, I am honored to have seen and participated in this new field of patient care.

Tactical medicine does not limit your ability to practice good medicine. It simply changes how you apply what you already know as you provide good patient care to the ill and injured without becoming a patient yourself. Tactical medics (medical doctors, physician assistants, or emergency medical technicians) must be well rounded, with the ability to apply a specific type of evaluation and care to each tactical situation they face. Although the tactical operators are generally healthy police officers, in many situations the suspects, hostages, and bystanders are certainly not, requiring providers who are skilled in both medical and trauma care.

Preparing for the Mission

Tactical training involves the completion of a 2-week police SWAT school and a 3-day tactical medical program and bimonthly tactical training with the team. The provider's participation in the SWAT school also fosters the camaraderie that is necessary in all successful units. Medically, the basic concepts of the ABCs are reviewed, and each provider masters advanced techniques in the control of bleeding and securing an emergent airway.

A significant philosophical difference in tactical medicine involves changing the emotional and tactical mind-sets of the operators and providers to keep them feel free to stray away from the ingrained ABC pattern of patient care. The introduction of the "care under fire" concept is critically important during the training of tactical medicine providers. This concept suggests that when a threat poses danger to you and the team, the best way to ensure your safety is to eliminate the threat and get the wounded to a place where they will receive proper care.

In order for this concept to be successful, all team members must carry a small "blowout" kit and be trained in controlling external *hemorrhage* and in performing basic airway/breathing techniques, which address the two primary causes of increased mortality in hostile situations. In addition, immediate tactical medical care must be in close proximity to those injured so that additional lifesaving measures can be quickly initiated. Providers should be trained in techniques that allow them to safely and rapidly extricate patients from immediate danger. In-depth education in tactical medical preplanning allows providers to recognize, evaluate, and solve many issues, even ones they haven't yet thought of, before they encounter those situations.

As a member of a police tactical team, I can report that operationally, teams' roles have been expanded into many dimensions, which, in turn, has required tactical medicine providers to incorporate new areas of patient care. We don't only respond to hostage situations or barricaded subjects, which was once our bread and butter. Currently, we are very active in asset protection and in conducting high-risk search or arrest warrants on armed individuals involved in selling illicit drugs, stealing weapons, and committing violent crimes. We have also been recruited by the U.S. Department of Homeland Security to assist in securing ports and waterways and in escorting high-value assets. All these operational platforms come with their own sets of potential challenges, which makes tactical medicine even more interesting.

Stories From the Field

One afternoon, the Special Investigations Unit asked our team to arrest a high-volume narcotics dealer who was known to be armed with a handgun and was due to make a delivery to several of his street-level peddlers that afternoon. The operational plan was to conduct a tactical vehicle takedown of the subject as he left his residence. During the execution of our plan, the dealer rammed several police vehicles in an attempt to flee in his vehicle but was subsequently stopped. As tactile officers approached him, he leaned forward and reached under his seat. Demonstrating great training and restraint, an officer fired a single shot that immediately incapacitated the subject. When officers removed him from the vehicle, they discovered that he had suffered a single exsanguinating supraclavicular gunshot wound. The patient was fully assessed, the bleeding was controlled, intravenous (IV) lines were established, and needle chest decompression was completed before local emergency medical services (EMS) arrived on the scene.

In another incident, an armed, mentally disturbed individual had barricaded himself inside a residence, and the uniform patrol division was trying to establish negotiations with him. Suddenly, our team came under a barrage of gunfire from the residence. Two officers were wounded in this exchange; one had an exsanguinating hemorrhage from a transected brachial artery injury. Thankfully, I was only 2 feet away and was able to control the hemorrhages from both wounds and extricate each officer from the dangerous area to awaiting EMS units. The bond that these two officers and I now share is beyond belief.

Jeffery G. Yates is a physician assistant in trauma surgery at Northfolk General Hospital, a level 1 trauma center in Northfolk, VA, and an Associate Professor with the Eastern Virginia Medical School (EVMS) PA program. A 2003 EVMS PA program graduate, he has been a Portsmouth Police Department SWAT medic since 1996. Prior to becoming a PA, he was a paramedic for 15 years.

Reprinted, with permission, from *PA Professional*, February 2012.

[CHAPTER 9]

Incentive

Success involves a course with many decisions along the way. Enjoy reading these physician assistant (PA) students' incentives toward their dream to become a PA.

PARISA SHABANZADEH, PA-S

In my aunt's eulogy, the orator stated, "On one's tombstone, it states one's birth date and one's death date. It does not matter when you were born or when you died, it is that dash in the middle that represents your whole life." I have adopted this philosophy wholeheartedly. Through my years, I have discovered that the most fulfilling way to spend my time is through community service. My goal to pursue a career as a physician assistant (PA) primarily stemmed from my commitment to volunteer work. As a permanent member of Alpha Gamma Sigma, an honors society that recognizes scholarship and promotes community service, I was honored with the President's Volunteer Service Award for my dedication to serving the community. Volunteering exposed me to many career paths that would fulfill my passion to help underserved low-income communities. However, when introduced to the PA profession and its philosophy and mission, I knew it was the perfect profession for me.

To gain knowledge of the responsibilities and qualities of a PA, I carried out extensive research, began shadowing a PA, and got accepted into the Los Angeles County + University of Southern California PA Helper Program. Under the guidance of a PA, I witnessed the skills and traits necessary to be an effective PA. One must be respectful, compassionate, able to relate to others, and able to communicate and educate efficiently and effectively while also capable of maintaining calm and collected demeanor under pressure.

Working in a doctor's office, I demonstrated and enhanced these same qualities on a daily basis. A few years before PA school, I met a patient who had been diagnosed with breast cancer. On removal of her breast, she was consumed with depression fueled by her "deformity," and although she was in much pain, she could not afford surgery. I comforted her and single-handedly had her surgery approved by Medi-Cal, thus giving her the ability to get the reconstructive surgery she needed. Most rewarding was when I aided in her postoperative care. Such events made me feel that with more education, experience, and resources, I would have the means to change lives.

Although my passion is healthcare, I received a BA in psychology. My background gave me the ability to aid patients psychologically and physically rather than simply objectively. I feel that it is crucial to treat patients as a whole. As a PA, I intend to educate patients on taking care of their health to minimize their visits and prevent disease, which will not only improve their physical well-being but also empower them.

It is the dash on one's tombstone that makes life worthwhile. My experience and research in the PA profession have made me understand and respect the role of PAs. In today's harsh economy, it is crucial that the PA profession exists to offer cost-effective healthcare. I believe that "the object of all education should be to increase the usefulness of man—usefulness to himself and others" and trust that my PA program will help me to accomplish this.

SARAH BROOME, PA-C

She was the first patient I assisted as a volunteer at Shriner's Hospital for Children. She was 6 years old, fidgeting with her full-body burn garment, and responding to questions with only head movements. As I spoke to her in both English and Spanish, she looked back puzzled. Although she must have been scared, the young girl did not cry or pull away as the therapist removed her garment to check her healing burns. She silently trusted us while we examined her patchwork of skin grafts. I learned that she had been medically evacuated from her remote village in Mexico to the closest pediatric burn hospital. Her pajamas had caught fire, burning her torso, arms, upper legs, and fingers. Her severely burned younger sister died in transport. Due to the cost of the trip, her family was unable to be with her. Despite her difficult situation, she demonstrated a courageous spirit. Looking into her eyes reaffirmed my interest in the healing process and intensified my desire to become a physician assistant (PA) in pediatric medicine.

The patients and staff at Shriners taught me about compassionate patient care, courage, and the opportunity for miracles in medicine. One such miracle involved a teenage boy who had suffered a severe spinal cord injury. Although the complications of his injury commonly resulted in paraplegia, I videotaped him as he broke into song, standing unsupported for the first time. It gave me great fulfillment to share in his success as I assisted him in relearning his walking gait. This young man and other brave patients taught me humility and strengthened my interest in the collaborative efforts in medicine.

Additionally, a Davis physical therapy clinic and a specialized pediatric research institute have exposed me to the challenges, responsibilities, and constant learning required of medical professionals. Outside of my work in pediatrics, older adults and their dedication to recovery also motivated me. After working in physical therapy for a year, I wanted to understand the patient's condition in greater depth. To broaden my exposure to the medical field, I began an internship with Dr. Hagerman, pediatrician and founder of the National Fragile X Foundation at the UC Davis Medical Investigation of Neurodevelopmental Disorders (MIND) Institute. I now have a full-time position and will increase my efforts with Dr. Hagerman's patients through assisting in the institute's clinic, research, and drug studies. I aspire to provide the same degree of commitment and hope that the MIND staff consistently gives to their patients and families.

I believe that becoming a PA will enable me to have a direct impact on the quality of patients' care. As an athlete and health advocate, I can work hard. I intend to meet challenges by maintaining openness to different working environments and patient backgrounds, offering compassionate care, and focusing on opportunities to improve my patient's condition.

LINDSEY STECKELBERG-ROBERTS, PA-S

Looking at the x-ray, I was amazed at the fact that I could see a coin inside my throat. I was 5 years old and, like any child, maintained the habit of placing indigestible objects into my mouth. After my sister tattled on me for swallowing the penny, my parents used a metal detector to determine its location before rushing me to the hospital. To their dismay, the x-ray showed the penny standing upright in my pharynx with the potential to fall flat and cause a blockage of my airway. While I was completely terrified, I was impressed with the fact that there was a "picture" of my insides (in which we could actually see President Lincoln's silhouette). This was the experience that caused me to repeatedly tell my mother, "I want to help people who are sick like I was!" Personal exposure to this unnerving event opened my eyes to the field of medicine.

Later in life I began volunteering at the local hospital. My first project was working with an autistic 5-year-old boy. While teaching him vital skills, I was able to sense that I was genuinely improving his life. To watch him advance and exemplify necessary social and attentive skills as a result of my assistance was the greatest compensation. Being in the hospital environment made me realize that many patients and families were in pain and bound by fear. They needed a listening ear and reassurance that things would be okay. If I could, I would listen to every person's story that stepped foot inside the hospital. I acknowledged that it was my duty to care for these individuals and put them at ease.

In another setting, I volunteered in the special care unit, where intensive care was administered. During my first shift, a patient lost his life, and it was my job to comfort his friends and relatives. Meanwhile, I was also making the waiting area comfortable for an elderly man who had been sleeping there for a week during his wife's recovery from a stroke. I have a passion for helping others, and becoming a PA would allow me to fulfill that dream. My level of determination and enthusiasm leaves no doubt in my mind that I will excel in my chosen field.

BREANNE STRENKOWSKI, PA-S

My life for the past 5 years has revolved around running. Everything, down to the mundane details of my life—when I eat, when I study, when I work, when I go to bed—is all determined by my running schedule. Everything I do, whether it is running 100-mile weeks or saying no to the spring-break Cabo trip, is part of a calculated plan that will take me to the next level in my running career. This obsession to perform at the highest level and to reach my full potential began in my freshman year in college and has molded me into the person I am today. My running career facilitated the development of discipline, diligence, and leadership. When my work ethic led to competing in the NCAA Cross Country

Championship in my freshman year, I became team captain for both University of California Santa Barbara's (UCSB) track and cross-country teams. This leadership role has taught me how to encourage and confront my peers while operating under the pressures of my coach's expectations of me and my team. These attributes have paid dividends in all aspects of my life, especially in my journey toward becoming a physician assistant (PA).

Running at the highest level requires a strict and healthy lifestyle: eating well, taking care of myself mentally and physically, and vigorous exercise. Everything must work in unison, at full output, in order to run a successful race. When I began running for UCSB, I quickly realized that I needed to fully immerse myself into the program if I ever wanted to tap into my full potential. I fell in love with biochemistry, biology, and physiology because they taught me how my body operates down to a molecular level. With an in-depth understanding of my physiology, I was able to fine-tune my preparation. I became infatuated with cooking, learning about nutrition, and optimal recovery. I learned to individualize and fine-tune my body through my diet and workouts. As a team captain, I have been passionate about teaching teammates how to get the most out of their bodies, whether it is through nutrition, training, recovery, or injury prevention. My love for physical well-being does not stop here because I will take my passion for human wellness into my career as a PA.

Numerous running-related injuries have landed me in the offices of dozens of physicians, physical therapists, and chiropractors. My job as a student athlete does not afford me the luxury of many other patients. Certain medications and time off from running are not paths I can travel lightly. Unfortunately, many of the professionals I worked with were either quick to write me a prescription or issue an ultimatum to quit running. It wasn't until I met Kathleen Pavel, a PA, that a healthcare professional finally worked with me to personalize my treatment to fit my running lifestyle. After hearing my symptoms and considering my sport, she explained her diagnosis in scientific terms and laid out the path to recovery considering my circumstances. She introduced me to the PA profession and inspired me to help individuals who are in unique situations and need individualized care.

Working with the developmentally disabled for Genesis also has helped me to realize this need for individualized care. Ann, a 61-year-old who is blind and mentally handicapped, is in a unique circumstance that requires personal care around the clock. When I started working with Ann,

I noticed that she used short phrases she learned as a child to help her remember how to do tasks such as walking up the stairs or showering. Rather than routinely delivering medications and tending to her physical needs, I work with the mind-set of helping Ann to do more for herself every day so that together we can achieve the ultimate goal of an increase in her confidence, independence, happiness, and healthy lifestyle. I push Ann to become more independent by teaching her to do her laundry, clean her dishes, tie her shoes, and cook. By my teaching Ann short phrases such as "Low and slow," she is able to remember how to stir a pot or mix up cookie dough. Three weeks after I taught Ann the phrase "Low and slow" while cooking, she repeated the phrase on her own. This memorable moment made me realize how much Ann had progressed during the time I worked with her. Helping Ann grow as a person has helped me to grow as a person. She taught me the valuable lessons of patience and compassion—new strengths that I will carry forward into my career.

After struggling through many injuries throughout my career, I realize the importance of an active and effective treatment. With my leadership and science background, I look forward to treating patients with a sense of urgency and proficiency. Through my experiences working and volunteering, I am prepared to begin my journey as a PA, where I will devote my career to helping patients quickly return to an active and healthy lifestyle so that their health is not the limiting factor in their journey to reach their full potential.

NESYAH SHAESTEH, PA-S

Involvement and familiarity with the healthcare field is something that I have been raised with when considering potential career options. As I gained more and more experience on the personal, academic, and professional levels, the question became not whether I would work in healthcare, but in what capacity I would do so. Because my oldest brother is a practicing dentist and my sister is a registered dietitian, in both cases I have witnessed firsthand the sacrifices made in the educational process, as well as the great rewards gained from working with patients. Based on years of exploration and self-examination, I have determined that a career as a physician assistant (PA) is the ideal choice for me as I improve health and overall quality of life.

Around the same time that I was observing the progress of my siblings in the medical field, I had an intense personal experience that inspired me greatly as well. One day, while sitting in the living room at home, my father instructed me to call 911. In a few minutes I was in a car following the ambulance that was taking him to the hospital. On arrival, I witnessed the sight of a medical team springing into action. Doctors, nurses, and, yes, PAs were all involved. In a heightened state of alert, I watched every move as they took my father's blood pressure and attached wires to his arms, legs, and chest for an electrocardiogram. Papers and test results flew out of machines. Results from his CT scan, MRI, and ECG were documented in his record. I remember this occasion as being extremely emotional for me, and yet I was mesmerized by the work of the team in the emergency room. I was amazed not only by their technical expertise but also by the care and concern they showed for my father and even for me as a family member. I couldn't believe that after doing so much to treat my father, they also had the time and ability to soothe and calm me as I looked on. It was truly inspiring. When things calmed down and I knew that my father would be okay, I experienced an epiphany in reflecting on what I had seen and felt. It was then and there that I knew that I would like to work as part of the same type of medical team that I had seen in the emergency room.

In recent years, I have explored my interest in healthcare both academically and in the working world. It was this powerful sense of drive that propelled me through a period when I took extended course loads in school, as many as 20 credits in a single semester, while simultaneously maintaining a full slate of volunteer work and extracurricular activities. While this seems daunting to think about in retrospect, it was completely invigorating at the time. I have found that I have deep reserves of energy when it comes to pursuing the things that genuinely interest me. Academically, my strongest passion and aptitude clearly were in the sciences. I took great interest in courses such as anatomy, physiology, microbiology, and general chemistry. I take this as an indication that I will always be naturally motivated to learn as much as possible both in school and as a future PA. Meanwhile, I put my growing scientific knowledge to work in the field by shadowing professionals such as Dr. Theodore Friedman, one of the prominent endocrinologists in the United States, and Dr. Farah Hekmat, a pediatrician. In the case of Dr. Friedman, I assisted in both the research lab and the treatment of patients in a clinical setting. This epitomized the varied sources of mental stimulation that I experienced and that thrilled me about the field. With both experiences, I began to gain a sense of my ability to work as part of a team.

It was at this time that I began to narrow my focus to the PA career specifically. The more I researched about the field, the more I realized that it perfectly suited my interest, abilities, and long-term goals. Working as a PA will enable me to enjoy a career in a field I love while also maintaining a sense of balance in my life. As I look forward to becoming a future wife and mother, I want to have the ability to balance work and family. I am confident that I can do this as a PA, gaining fulfillment from my career while also being available to spend time with my family.

Pursuing a career as a PA is my attempt to "have it all"—to attain my childhood dream of working in the medical field while also having a family of my own. From the time I was very young, and from the time I was exposed to the incredible work of an emergency room medical team, I have envisioned myself working in such an environment. I have thrived on great challenges in the past and will continue to do so in the future. With the benefit of a good education from a strong PA program, I know that I will take an important step toward the realization of my goals.

[CHAPTER 10]

Inspirational Leaders: A Collection of Personal Professional Biographies

Having a mentor who inspires you to strive toward your desired professional goals may be one of life's greatest gifts. Finding that person who has the time to share his or her experiences with you one on one can be difficult. I have chosen unique, hard-working, and successful physician assistants (PAs) who were kind enough to share their professional life story and give advice. My hope is that learning more about these inspiring PAs' involvement in the academic, managerial, and leadership roles will challenge you to become similarly involved in shaping the future of PAs in the healthcare system.

1. Andrew J. Rodican, PA-C, business owner and author of *The Ultimate Guide to Getting into Physician Assistant School* and *How to "Ace" the Physician Assistant School Interview.*

2. William C. Kohlhepp, DHSc, PA-C, past president of the American Academy of Physician Assistants (AAPA) and current associate dean of the Quinnipiac University School of Health Sciences.

3. Robert Sammartano, PA-C, pediatric surgery, program director, postgraduate residency in surgery for physician assistants, and past president of the American Association of Surgical Physician Assistants (AASPA).

4. Joyce Nichols, PA-C, first woman to be formally educated as a physician assistant (PA) and the first African-American woman to practice as a PA. Biography by Janette Rodrigues from *PA Professional Magazine*.

PROFESSIONAL BIOGRAPHY OF ANDREW J. RODICAN, PA-C

Jessica Rodriguez Ohanesian, MS, PA-C

Andrew Rodican, PA-C, has had an impact on aspiring physician assistants (PAs) throughout his career. I first learned of him through his self-published book, *The Ultimate Guide to Getting into Physician Assistant School*, which was later republished by the McGraw-Hill. His second book, *How to "Ace" the Physician Assistant School Interview*, was self-published in 2011. He is an inspiration both as an author and as a PA, and I am honored to write about his life and professional achievements.

Andy was first introduced to medicine in the 1970s while serving as a Navy corpsman. During those 4 years, his job duties reflected that of a midlevel healthcare provider. After an honorable discharge from the Navy, he worked as an emergency room technician at Yale–New Haven Hospital, and there he became familiar with the career opportunities of a PA. The PA profession was a natural transition from his prior experiences and required only 2 years of additional schooling. He also chose this career path because he enjoyed the challenging and rewarding role PAs play in the healthcare system.

In 1994, Andy graduated from Yale University's School of Medicine Physician Associate Program. He was the recipient of their Medical Writing Award and served on the admissions committee both as a student and as an alumni member. In 1996, he published his first book and formed his first company, AJR Associates, both of which were focused on assisting PA school applicants through the admissions process. The epiphany behind his book idea for *The Ultimate Guide to Getting into Physician Assistant School* came about during a phone conversation with a friend in which Andy expressed disappointment in meeting excellent PA school applicants who had failed to gain acceptance into a PA school. They had made small yet critical mistakes in their essay or interview that had cost them their acceptance.

His friend simply stated, "You should write a book about it." These candidates were lacking an educational mentoring resource to guide them through the application process, and his book met that need.

Andy's favorite PA student rotation was in the field of cardiovascular surgery. He experienced the stress and excitement of the operating room and cultivated skills in taking care of complicated patients postoperatively. This rotation resulted in his first job as a cardiovascular surgery PA. It took 3 months of extreme dedication and hard work before he gained some sense of comfort and confidence, but he went on to become the chief PA and remained in this subspecialty for 3 years.

Occupational medicine was his next subspecialty calling, and he remained there for 7 years. In 1997, he opened a workers' compensation clinic for his employer at the Mohegan Sun Casino in Uncasville, CT. The Mohegan Sun is the second largest casino in the world, employing up to 10,000 people. Until that time, the casino sent all of its employees to the local emergency room for work-related injuries. This was extremely expensive and inefficient. The clinic Andy started remains in place today.

In 2002, Andy experienced a life-changing and career-altering event: He suffered a heart attack. Before this event, he had undergone excessive weight gain, which led to diabetes, hypertension, obstructive sleep apnea, and acid reflux disease. His firsthand experience with the negative and potentially deadly effects of obesity caused him to open a weight-loss clinic at the cardiology practice for which he worked. After losing 50 pounds, he was able to slowly taper off all his medications and his sleep apnea machine. His successes inspired many of his patients and led him to his next subspecialty and current practice in bariatric medicine.

In 2009, Andy became one of four PAs in the country to pass the certification examination and receive a Certification of Advanced Training in Bariatric Medicine from the American Board of Obesity Medicine (ABOM). He is the owner and founder of Medical Weight Loss Centers in East Haven, CT. What he enjoys most about his current role is being able to take patients off prescription medications and watch how proper diet and lifestyle changes can cure disease.

His best advice for a new graduate PA is this: First, follow your passion. Second, keep an open mind because you never know what opportunities are in store for your future. Lastly, don't chase after money or prestige; chase your passion, and everything else will follow.

PROFESSIONAL BIOGRAPHY OF WILLIAM "BILL" C. KOHLHEPP, DHSC, PA-C

Jessica Rodriguez Ohanesian, MS, PA-C

William "Bill" C. Kohlhepp, DHSc, PA-C, has been a devoted leader for the physician assistant (PA) profession since 1977, involved in clinical practice, research, publications, professorship, and various leadership positions, including serving as president of the American Academy of Physician Assistants (AAPA) in 1999–2000. He also obtained a doctor of health sciences degree from Nova Southeastern University in 2007. Bill currently serves as the associate dean of the School of Health Sciences at Quinnipiac University and is the secretary and treasurer of the Physician Assistant Education Association (PAEA). He exemplifies a PA committed to educational achievement and leadership.

After completing an undergraduate degree in biology from the University of Connecticut in 1974, Bill maintained an interest in medicine but decided against medical school. His college roommate went straight to PA school and provided some insight into the career of physician assistant. What captivated Bill's interest most was the meaningful role a PA plays in the delivery of healthcare and the significant relationship a PA has with his or her patients.

In 1979, Bill was part of the third graduating class of Rutgers University/University of Medicine and Dentistry of New Jersey Allied Health Program. As a student, he contributed in the formation of the Physician Assistant Student Society of New Jersey and the New Jersey State Society of Physician Assistants. This began his relationship with the American Academy of Physician Assistants (AAPA). At that time, it was illegal to work as a PA in the state of New Jersey unless you were practicing in a federal agency, such as the Veterans Administration. "Without the challenge of being in a state where PAs could not practice, I would not have understood the strength one gains as a professional when working together with other members of that profession to accomplish goals," states Bill. "It truly was the spark that has led me to a lifetime of involvement in PA professional organizations." In 1977, he attended his first AAPA conference and realized the importance of networking and meeting new people. In 1978, the Student Academy of the AAPA appointed him to serve as a liaison to the Association of Physician Assistant Programs (now PAEA).

Fresh out of school, Bill relocated to New Haven, CT, to work as a PA in the Emergency Department at Yale–New Haven Hospital. This job combined both clinical practice and research through Yale University, which led to his authorship of a publication in the *New England Journal of Medicine* in 1982, "A Protocol for Selecting Patients with Extremity Injuries Who Need X-Rays." After 4 years' experience in this setting, he decided to pursue a different area of concentration.

In 1983, Bill chose family practice as his next subspecialty, where he worked full time clinically with three physicians and two other PAs. Two years later, within the same company, Bill was chosen to manage and work at a new satellite clinic this practice had opened. The leadership skills he acquired working alongside AAPA better prepared him for the managerial role he would assume. During this dual clinic/management role, he spent time caring for employees with occupational injuries. This developed a new subspecialty interest that would later affect his career. Financial circumstances and healthcare model inadequacies caused him to pursue other employment.

Bill found his next job as a healthcare operations manager after seeing an advertisement in the newspaper. It was highly competitive, but he credits this job opportunity to networking and name recognition via his service with the AAPA. From 1989 to 1996, he served as an operations manager for the outpatient occupational medicine practice at the Hospital of Saint Raphael. During this time, he continued part-time clinical work treating hospital employees with occupational injuries. He oversaw all medical employees, including physical therapists, occupational therapists, and clinicians. He wrote a business plan covering systems to run the practice, billing, and eventually, plans to expand the practice. When he stepped in as operations manager, this practice consisted of one physician and two nurses providing services only to hospital employees. When he left, the practice employed four physicians and six PAs and provided services to over 300 companies.

During his time at the Hospital of Saint Raphael, a friend and occupational therapist left her job to teach at Quinnipiac University. Bill expressed his interest in teaching and requested that she contact him regarding PA professorship opportunities. He thought, "I can make a difference to help the reputation and growth of the profession one person at a time, or I can teach and instill values into the future generation of PAs." A year later he received a call, seized the opportunity, and transitioned into his next career opportunity—PA professorship.

Bill's work at Quinnipiac University began in 1996 as an academic coordinator, and he remained in this role for 6 years. His greatest reward was watching students transition from the classroom setting into their career and later into leadership positions within the profession. In 2002, he was promoted to associate director of the physician assistant program, and in 2007, he became director. He has a wide range of responsibilities, including involvement with admissions, administration, disciplinary action, management, and education. He now serves as the associate dean of the Quinnipiac University School of Health Sciences.

"When you do something, get involved" is the driving statement that has pushed Bill to remain involved in PA leadership. Bill's fight for PAs to have practicing rights in New Jersey started a cascade of service with the AAPA that has continued for over 30 years. He began at the committee-service level and progressed to a house of delegates officer: secretary (1991–1992), second vice speaker (1992–1993), two terms as first vice speaker (1993–1994, 1994–1995), three terms as speaker (1995–1996, 1996–1997, 1997–1998), and president-elect (1998–1999). Bill then served as the AAPA president from 1999 to 2000, the highest nationwide honor for a PA. Following his term as president, he served a year as chairman of the AAPA board of directors/immediate past president (2000–2001). He later served a 6-year term as AAPA's liaison to the American Medical Association. Bill has served in the AAPA house of delegates as either a delegate or alternate since 1979. What he enjoys most about his involvement with the AAPA is the ability to make a difference and the abundance of friends and colleagues he has made across the nation.

Of the many honors and awards Bill received throughout his career, there are three of which he is particularly proud. First, he was the first-ever PA to be awarded the Distinguished Alumnus Award from the School of Health Related Professions at the University of Medicine and Dentistry of New Jersey in 1999. Second, in 2009, he received an honorary doctor of humane letters award from AT Still University in Mesa, AZ. And third, he received the James Marshall Award for Outstanding Service to Quinnipiac University in 2010. The most rewarding PA role he has undertaken has been as a member of the committee formed to write and define PA competencies, which include medical knowledge, interpersonal and communication skills, patient care, professionalism, practice-based learning and improvement, and systems-based practice. The purpose of the competencies is to communicate to the PA profession and the public the capabilities and expectations of PAs.

Bill has two favorite quotes:

"Listen to the patient, for he is trying to give you the diagnosis."
—Sir William Osler

"If you're doing something you care that much about, and you believe in its purpose deeply enough, then it is impossible to imagine not trying to make it great."
—Jim Collins, in his book, From Good to Great

Bill's advice for new graduate PAs as they start their careers is "Be passionate, get involved, and make a difference in giving back to your physician assistant community. This is not a just a job, this is a profession, and you will get as much out of this profession as you put into it. The acquired extracurricular skills you will gain through giving back will build your confidence and will open doors for future opportunities."

PROFESSIONAL BIOGRAPHY OF ROBERT SAMMARTANO, RPA-C

Jessica Rodriguez Ohanesian, MS, PA-C

Robert "Bob" Sammartano, RPA-C, works as a surgical physician assistant (PA) clinically, a postgraduate residency program director educationally, a policy maker as a house of delegates officer, and an organizational leader as president of the American Association of Surgical Physician Assistants (AASPA). So many accomplishments, yet his PA career began later in life, following 19 years working in surgical research. He infuses enthusiasm about the PA profession into everyone around him, and his story will surely inspire you.

In 1972, Bob graduated from Fordham University with a BS in biology. From 1972 to 1991, he worked as a research associate with Dr. Scott Boley, a world-renowned pediatric surgeon and professor of surgery and pediatrics at Montefiore Medical Center–Albert Einstein College of Medicine in New York City. For the first 11 years, he also worked side by side with Mr. Michael Sheran, RPA-C, the first pediatric surgical PA in the nation. In the laboratory, Bob implemented research protocols to study vascular disorders of the intestines. He also worked clinically, assisting in the interpretation of angiograms and studying data from patients with vascular disorders such as acute mesenteric ischemia and vascular ectasias of the colon.

Bob was at Montefiore 4 years before the postgraduate surgery PA residency program graduated its first class. As a result, he observed first-hand the development of the surgical PA profession. Bob witnessed the physician-PA partnership while working alongside Dr. Boley and Michael Sheran. Michael passed away in 1987 after a long bout with leukemia, and shortly thereafter, Bob applied to Yale's PA program, in part to follow in Michael's footsteps. At the age of 41, Bob started PA school. Like Bob, many of his classmates had prior careers, yet he felt that his work and life experience had best prepared him to work as a PA and provided him with a sense of direction as to his selection of a subspecialty.

In 1993, Bob graduated from Yale University's School of Medicine Physician Associate Program with honors. Because of his friendship and prior work history with Dr. Boley, Bob seemed destined to go into pediatric surgery. He completed the 15-month postgraduate residency in surgery at Montefiore Medical Center–Albert Einstein College of Medicine. Clara Vanderbilt, RPA-C, the PA who "put the face of surgical PAs on the map" further inspired his calling for surgery. Clara trained at Duke University with Dr. Eugene Stead, founder of the PA profession. She was one of the first four PA surgical residents employed at Montefiore, and she helped to establish the first PA surgical postgraduate residency in the country. This same residency accelerated Bob's comfort level with patient care and helped him to transition into his first job.

In 1994, Bob began working with Dr. Boley as a pediatric surgical PA at Montefiore Medical Center. He has been the senior surgical PA there for the past two decades. "Think and act" is a favorite motto of Bob because he enjoys the decision making required during surgery. Bob loves working in pediatrics because he enjoys working with families and offering hope. He lets his pediatric patients know that they are not alone and often encourages them with a success story from one of his previous patients who had similar medical concerns. Bob states, "If the problem is caught early, pediatric surgery is extremely rewarding because one surgery has the ability to effect positive change or prolong life."

Bob became the program director for the PA postgraduate surgical residency at Montefiore in 2003. His responsibilities in this role include interviewing possible candidates, preparing the didactic course, giving lectures, arranging for required certifications for students, teaching hands-on workshops, and working clinically as a teacher and role model. Bob also travels locally in the New York metropolitan area to lecture at undergraduate PA programs, bringing both his experience in pediatric surgery and the merits of postgraduate training in surgery to first- and second-year students. His greatest reward is receiving letters from past students thanking him for such a high-quality learning experience and updating him on their professional successes.

Bob's various roles in AASPA have included president (2010–2012) and fellow and director at large (2003–2008). The AASPA supports the surgical PA profession through marketing, offering continuing medical education (CME) specific to surgery, assisting with professional issues (such as credentialing), and providing a forum for networking. This results in improved patient care and safety, enhanced revenue streams, decreased physician workloads, increased visibility for the surgical PA profession, and increased employment and compensation for PAs. The most enjoyable part of Bob's involvement with AASPA is his ability to make an impact. Bob states, "It is gratifying to make change and to make change for the better."

Bob defines leadership as "the consequence of being truly enamored with what one has chosen as a career. It is the passing of the baton from colleagues who have run the same race, recognizing [that] you can be part of where the PA profession needs to go." While at Yale, Bob was the student representative to the Connecticut Association of Physician Assistants (ConnAPA), a constituent organization of the American Academy of Physician Assistants (AAPA). He continued his affiliation with AAPA as a member over the years and encourages PAs to be AAPA members because "the AAPA has political clout by membership numbers. AAPA effects your life as a PA. It influences how you practice, where you practice and helps to enrich your scope of practice as a PA. This organization is the voice for the PA profession at the national level, and an important organization to support." Since 2007, Bob has been the chief delegate of surgery for the AAPA house of delegates. Bob's drive for leadership is summarized in his statement, "If you believe in what you do, pick up the baton and look for someone to pass it to. The key is keeping the PA profession moving forward. You cannot spell 'apathy' without PA. Having a career, good salary, home, vacation plans, etc. makes us all comfortable. When someone taps you on the shoulder urging you to lead, be receptive and act. The obsolete thinking of 'medicine versus surgery' must disappear. We all are PAs with common goals that need to be obtained. Our differences in solving problems should not be barriers but options for solution."

Bob believes if he cannot infuse his enthusiasm into anyone, and especially a PA willing to listen, then he has not fulfilled his responsibilities to the profession. "If you love what you do, don't just let it lay fallow. Teach someone something every day. Small steps like that give the PA profession growth and energy."

PROFESSIONAL BIOGRAPHY OF JOYCE CLAYTON NICHOLS, PA-C

Janette Rodrigues, *PA Professional Magazine*

Joyce Clayton Nichols grew up on her family's farm in the gently rolling hills of central North Carolina. There they grew cash crops such as tobacco and wheat and raised some livestock. In the early twentieth century, one out of every seven farmers in the United States was African American. But during the same period, millions of African Americans left the South for new opportunities in cities in the North and West, such as New York, Chicago, and Los Angeles, and to escape oppressive Jim Crow laws. Her parents, though, decided to stay in Person County and raise their children on the land they fought to keep. Today, there are fewer than 18,000 African-American-owned farms in the country and fewer than 3,000 in North Carolina. In an "endangered" profession, the African-American farmer is quickly becoming extinct. Yet the Clayton family stuck it out. "We still own our family farm," she said recently, a note of pride in her voice. "We had a lot of fun there; I mean, we also worked hard because we would get up early in the morning to do whatever we had to do on the farm, and then we went to school. When we came home, we did whatever we had to get done."

Determination is a way of life for Nichols. It's what got her through the long, backbreaking days that come with farming. It's what got her through high school. It's what got her into, and through, the licensed practical nursing program at Durham Technical Community College. It's what helped her earn a place on staff of the Duke University Medical Center Cardiac Care Unit. And it's what led her, an African-American woman, working in the racially polarized South in late 1960s, to fiercely lobby the university to let her into the then all-male physician assistant (PA) program.

"I applied three times before I was accepted into the PA program," recalled Nichols, the first woman to be formally educated as a PA. "It was a male program, and I wasn't a military corpsman. The PA program was not for females, and female 'life expectancy' in the profession was low because the belief was that a female would start having babies and it would not be productive."

In 1968, she successfully argued her way into the program after convincing PA profession luminaries to take a chance on her: Eugene Stead, Jr., MD, founder of the PA profession and the Duke PA program concept; Harvey Estes, MD, the first chairman of the Department of Community Health Sciences at Duke; Robert Howard, MD, the Duke PA program's first full-time medical and program director; and Jim Mau, chief administrator for the Department of Medicine at Duke. (Duke Medical School did not admit its first African American until 1963.)

Rough Beginnings

The men overseeing the PA program didn't make it easy on Nichols. "Jim Mau came up to me on a Friday afternoon and told me that I had been accepted and that I had to report to class at 8 o'clock that Monday morning in the trailer," she said. "And I was scheduled to do evenings as a nurse, but I wouldn't have gotten out of class until 4 o'clock in the afternoon." A sympathetic nursing supervisor made sure that Nichols was able to stay in class the required hours before she started her evening shift in the CCU. "I have a tendency to be just as alley [cat] as anybody else, and I went off in the classroom and said that everybody there had an area of expertise, and we can work together to get through this," Nichols said. So every Wednesday, she and her classmates would meet for a study group. First, it was at a pub close to the Duke campus. The study group eventually migrated to her house. "We made a pact that everybody in our class would graduate on time." They supported her, and she supported them, and each did their fair share of tutoring the others. Things were falling into place. In December 1969, in the middle of her first year, a fire swept through her home. She and husband, Mike, and children, Will, 12, Le Von, 9, and Melita, 5, lost everything they owned, everything they had worked for. While no one was injured—she was in class, her husband at work, and the children at school—it was devastating. She decided to drop out of the program so that she could pick up some overtime to help her family get back on its feet. But her classmates wouldn't let her. "Those guys got together and sold tickets for a dance. They made enough money for us to buy furniture, clothing, and toys for my children for Christmas. I still have the tin box they put the money in and gave to me in 1969."

The 12 members of Nichols's class supported each other; they were a cohesive unit, and she was one of them. "The thing I'm most proud of accomplishing is developing a camaraderie with my classmates, even though it started out rocky, all of us were able to end up as a cohesive group," Nichols said. "We respected each other, and we looked out for each other. There is no way to explain what those first 3 months were like compared to the rest of the 21 months I spent with those guys. It was just unreal."

"And I don't have words to express it. They were a group of good guys after we got our differences taken care of." All the members of her class graduated and went on to practice as PAs.

Cardiology versus. General Practice

When Nichols was going through the PA program, she planned to become a PA in cardiology. She enjoyed being a cardiac care nurse, so it made sense for her to specialize in cardiology. She even did one of her clinical rotations in it. The other clinical rotation was in general practice with a rural family doctor, and it changed her life. The time she spent treating patients in Garland, NC, brought home some truths for her. "I realized then that I wanted to do internal medicine," Nichols said. "The general practitioner I worked for, Amos Johnson, his medical records were lousy, but he knew every one of his patients by name and their medical history. He had a young man, who he had trained, who could do anything. He could set broken legs and suture lacerations when they came in, and I fell in love with that and doing health education. And not only did Dr. Johnson own the clinic, but he owned the pharmacy as well." All of which appealed to the independent-minded daughter of a farmer. She also had firsthand knowledge of the difficulties of obtaining adequate healthcare in rural America.

During this time, the American Academy of Physician Assistants (AAPA) was being organized. PA William Stanhope, the academy's first president, gave Nichols, then a PA student, the job of writing the first draft of the organization's bylaws. She was elected to serve as a director at large on the AAPA board of directors in 1971. She and Prentiss Harrison, the first African-American PA, worked closely with PAs Earl Echard, John Davis, and Steve Turnipseed to establish AAPA's Minority Affairs Committee in the early 1970s. They also helped the profession gain acceptance among African-American physicians.

Prior to graduation, she met with Estes to discuss her employment plans. The PA profession was still finding its way, and it was difficult enough to help find jobs for white male graduates, much less an African-American female. Estes asked her what she wanted to do if she had the choice. "I told him that I wanted to have a rural health clinic. I told him about the difficulties people like my grandmother and other family members had because there was no place for them to go for preventive care."

Nichols credits Estes with helping her secure the funding to open what would become one of the first rural satellite health clinics in the nation. She was still a student when she met with clinic board members and advisors to conduct a health survey of the patients the facility would serve. When she graduated from the Duke PA program in 1970, the clinic was set up in the basement of a Baptist church and ready for her to start work in Rougemont, NC.

Taking the Salty with the Sweet

Nichols, friends and colleagues joke about her sometimes brusk, tell-it-like-it-is manner. "Joyce is the type of person who doesn't care what color you are; she will curse you out and she is the same when it comes to helping you," said PA Earl Echard, a long-time friend. "She thrives on things that are difficult. She has taken on things through the years that have been monumental that a lot of people have shied away from."

Born and raised not far from Rougemont, Nichols was not naive about how to get the white community on her side in the racially segregated area. "The thing that made me excited about going to work every day was home visits," she said, adding it helped her gain acceptance as a clinician in the white community.

"I made friends with the mail man, and through him I learned about one of the influential families in the area. This was a well-off family, and they were big landowners. The matriarch of the family had severe corns and calluses on her feet. I would go to that lady's home and soak her feet in water and manually take a scalpel and remove the corns and calluses off her feet. She was able to walk without a walker and wear her pretty shoes, and I was the best thing since sliced bread. And because of the pull her family had, it was automatic that I was accepted."

Another wealthy family donated land so that the clinic could build a proper facility because it had outgrown the church. By 1972, though, the external funding for the clinic began to dry up. She and Estes approached Lincoln Hospital, now Lincoln Health Center, which primarily served Durham's African-American community, to take over the clinic. Lincoln agreed, and Nichols began to split her time between the rural clinic and one operated by Lincoln in Durham public housing.

"So I was working two jobs—teaching classes in physician diagnosis at Duke Monday, Wednesday, and Friday and going out to the clinic in Rougemont at 10:30 a.m. on Monday, Wednesday and Friday. And Tuesdays and Thursdays I was at the [public housing] clinic until the load got too heavy, and I couldn't do both." Echard, who was a student when he first met Nichols, took over the Durham clinic after he graduated from the Duke PA program in 1973.

She took on more and more responsibilities as a PA educator and leader. She helped found the North Carolina Academy of Physician Assistants and served on its board of directors. She acted as a preceptor and taught as an adjunct faculty member in Duke's Department of Community and Family Medicine, yet Nichols refused to give up the rural clinic. "I loved my rural folk," she said. "And I understood their need for healthcare—preventive healthcare—so I would be there, and I would even do an evening clinic so that they could leave the field and come right on to the clinic."

Looking Back

Four decades have passed since she convinced the founders of the PA profession to let her through the door. (Some would say that she kicked it in.) She has taught and mentored generations of PAs from all walks of life. "Joyce has done so much, and she is such a humble person," said PA Barbara Bennett, a long-time friend. "She has been a mentor to so many people and been there for so many people. She encouraged you to continue your education, look beyond the general expectations and think outside the box. All the PAs who know Joyce respect her and love her. Some may have feared her because if you are wrong, she is going to let you know you are wrong, and she is not going to support you, and she is going to let you know what to do to rectify it."

Bennett added that her friend, mentor, and "big sister" has never been about the almighty dollar. "She has always wanted to help people be the best they could. Did you know in the summertime she would have this teaching program for middle school kids from Durham? She would take them to the beach for good behavior and academics, and being mediocre was not good enough to get to go on those trips."

AAPA President-elect Robert Wooten believes that Nichols had a vision for the profession. "She understood the hard work that it took to get into PA school and to successfully complete the program," he said. "She encouraged us to mentor other students along the way. She understood the obstacles that were out there facing PAs and encouraged others to overcome those obstacles. Joyce does not accept excuses or lack of effort."

Nichols retired from Lincoln Health Center in 1995, but she will never fully retire from the PA profession. "I've had a wonderful career, where I enjoyed what I was doing. I was able to be a clinician, a PA educator. When a college or university wanted to start a PA program, I went with [former Duke PA Program Director Bob] Howard to the sites to look at the programs.

And whatever task she took on or was given, she had the determination to see it through—whether it was rushing a patient to a clinic in the back of a flat-bed truck on back country roads or becoming the first female PA."

Reprinted, with permission, from *PA Professional*, September 2010.

APPENDIX A

Physician Assistant Schools

This information is provided by the Accreditation Review Commission on Education for the Physician Assistant (ARC-PA) at www.arc-pa.com/acc_programs/index.html and was last updated on April 12, 2013.

State	Accredited Program
AL	University of South Alabama www.southalabama.edu/alliedhealth/pa/
AL	University of Alabama at Birmingham www.uab.edu/cds/academic/graduate/spa
AR	Harding University www.harding.edu/PAprogram/
AR	University of Arkansas (provisional[†]) www.uams.edu/chrp/pa/
AZ	Arizona School of Health Sciences (probation*) www.atsu.edu/ashs/NA SCHOOL OF HEALTH SCIENCES 5850 E. S
AZ	Midwestern University (Glendale) www.midwestern.edu/Course_Catalog_Home/Glendale_AZ_Campus_/College_of_Health_Sciences/Physician_Assistant_Program.html
AZ	Northern Arizona University (provisional[†]) http://nau.edu/CHHS/PA/Program/
CA	Loma Linda University www.llu.edu/allied-health/sahp/pa/index.page
CA	Riverside Community College (probation*) www.rccd.edu/services/admissions/Pages/index.aspx

(Continued)

State	Accredited Program
CA	Samuel Merritt College www.samuelmerritt.edu/physician_assistant
CA	San Joaquin Valley College (probation*) www.sjvc.edu/program/Physician_Assistant/
CA	Stanford University http://pcap.stanford.edu/
CA	Touro University, California www.tu.edu/
CA	University of California-Davis www.ucdmc.ucdavis.edu/fnppa/
CA	University of Southern California (LA) http://keck.usc.edu/Education/Academic_Department_and_ Divisions/Physician_Assistant_Program.aspx
CA	Western University of Health Sciences www.westernu.edu/allied-health
CO	Red Rocks Community College www.rrcc.edu/pa/
CO	University of Colorado www.ucdenver.edu/academics/colleges/medicalschool/education/ degree_programs/PAProgram/Pages/Home.aspx
CT	University of Bridgeport (provisional†) www.bridgeport.edu/academics/graduate/pa/default.aspx
CT	Quinnipiac University www.quinnipiac.edu/x781.xml
CT	Yale University School of Medicine www.paprogram.yale.edu/
DC	George Washington University www.gwu.edu/~gwu_pa
DC	Howard University (probation*) www.cpnahs.howard.edu/AHS/Pa/Introduction.htm
FL	Barry University (D) www.barry.edu/pa/

State	Accredited Program
FL	Miami-Dade College www.mdc.edu/medical
FL	Keiser University www.keiseruniversity.edu/graduateschool/PA/
FL	Nova Southeastern University, Ft. Lauderdale www.nova.edu/pa
FL	Nova Southeastern University, Jacksonville www.nova.edu/pa/Jacksonville
FL	Nova Southeastern University, Southwest Florida www.nova.edu/panaples
FL	Nova Southeastern University, Orlando www.nova.edu/pa/Orlando
FL	South University, Tampa www.southuniversity.edu/tampa/physician-assistant-studies-degree-ms-149412.aspx
FL	University of Florida http://medinfo.ufl.edu/pa/
GA	Emory University www.emorypa.org/
GA	Georgia Health Sciences University www.georgiahealth.edu/alliedhealth/pa/index.html
GA	Mercer University http://cophs.mercer.edu/pa.htm
GA	South University www.southuniversity.edu/
IA	Des Moines University www.dmu.edu/pa/
IA	University of Iowa http://paprogram.medicine.uiowa.edu/
ID	Idaho State University www.isu.edu/PAprog/

(Continued)

State	Accredited Program
IL	John H. Stroger Hospital of Cook County/Malcolm X (Chicago City-Wide/Cook County from 1988–1992) (probation*) www.ccc.edu/colleges/malcolm-x/programs/pages/physician-assistant-associate-in-applied-science.aspx
IL	Midwestern University (Downers-Grove) www.midwestern.edu/Programs_and_Admission/IL_Physician_Assistant_Studies.html
IL	Northwestern University www.familymedicine.northwestern.edu/pa_program
IL	Rosalind Franklin University of Medicine (formerly Finch) www.rosalindfranklin.edu/
IL	Rush University (provisional†) www.rushu.rush.edu/servlet/Satellite?c=RushUnivLevel2Page&cid=1252283770149&pagename=Rush/RushUnivLevel2Page/Level_2_College_GME_CME_Page
IL	Southern Illinois University http://paprogram.siuc.edu/
IN	Butler University www.butler.edu/cophs
IN	Indiana State University (provisional†) www.indstate.edu/pa/
IN	Indiana University School of Health and Rehabilitation Sciences (provisional†) www.shrs.iupui.edu/health_sciences/degrees/physician_assistant.html
IN	University of St. Francis (Fort Wayne) www.sf.edu/sf/physician-assistant/ms-entry
KS	Wichita State University http://chp.wichita.edu/pa
KY	University of the Cumberlands http://gradweb.ucumberlands.edu/medicine/mpas
KY	University of Kentucky (D) www.mc.uky.edu/PA/
LA	Our Lady of the Lake‡ (provisional†) www.ololcollege-edu.org/content/admissions-academic-programs-physician-assistant-studies

State	Accredited Program
LA	Louisiana State University—Shreveport www.medcom.lsuhscshreveport.edu/ah/page.php?id=23
LA	Louisiana State University - New Orleans (provisional[†]) alliedhealth.lsuhsc.edu/pa/
MA	Bay Path College (provisional[†]) www.baypath.edu/GraduateProgram/GraduateDegrees/ MSPhysicianAssistant.aspx
MA	Massachusetts College of Pharmacy (Boston) www.mcphs.edu/
MA	Northeastern University www.northeastern.edu/bouve/pa/
MA	Springfield College www.spfldcol.edu/
MA	Tufts University (provisional[†]) http://publichealth.tufts.edu/Academics/Physician-Assistant-Program
MD	Anne Arundel Community College www.arc-pa.com/acc_programs/www.aacc.edu/physassist
MD	Towson University CCBC—Essex www.ccbcmd.edu/
MD	University of Maryland Eastern Shore www.umes.edu/pa
ME	University of New England www.une.edu/chp/pa
MI	Central Michigan University www.chp.cmich.edu/
MI	Grand Valley State University www.gvsu.edu/pa
MI	University of Detroit/Mercy http://healthprofessions.udmercy.edu/programs/paprogram/index.php
MI	Wayne State University www.pa.cphs.wayne.edu/
MI	Western Michigan University www.wmich.edu/hhs/pa

(Continued)

State	Accredited Program
MN	Saint Catherine University (provisional[†]) www.stkate.edu/academic/mpas/
MN	Augsburg College www.augsburg.edu/pa
MS	Mississippi College (provisional[†]) www.mc.edu/academics/departments/pa/
MO	Saint Louis University www.slu.edu/x2348.xml
MO	Missouri State University (formerly SWMS) www.missouristate.edu/pas
MT	Rocky Mountain College www.rocky.edu/academics/academic-programs/graduate-programs/mpas/index.php
NC	Duke University Medical Center http://pa.mc.duke.edu/
NC	Campbell University (provisional[†]) www.campbellpharmacy.net/academics/graduate/mspas/index.html
NC	East Carolina University www.ecu.edu/pa
NC	Elon University (provisional[†]) www.elon.edu/e-web/academics/pa/
NC	Methodist University www.methodist.edu/paprogram
NC	Wake Forest University (Bowman Gray) www1.wfubmc.edu/PAProgram
NC	Wingate University (D) http://pa.wingate.edu/
ND	University of North Dakota www.med.und.edu/physicianassistant/
NE	Union College www.ucollege.edu/pa
NE	University of Nebraska www.unmc.edu/alliedhealth/pa

State	Accredited Program
NH	Franklin Pierce University www.franklinpierce.edu/academics/gradstudies/programs_of_study/ master_physician_assistant.htm
NH	MCPHS University (Manchester/Worcester) www.mcphs.edu/
NJ	MCPHS University (Manchester/Worcester) www.shu.edu/
NJ	UMDNJ (formerly UMDNJ/Rutgers University) www2.umdnj.edu/paweb/
NM	University of New Mexico (probation*) http://hsc.unm.edu/
NM	University of St. Francis www.stfrancis.edu/pa/index.htm
NV	Touro University Las Vegas www.tun.touro.edu/
NY	Albany Medical College www.amc.edu/pa?
NY	CCNY Sophie Davis School of Biomedical Education http://med.cuny.edu/
NY	Clarkson University (provisional[†]) www.clarkson.edu/pa/
NY	Cornell University www.med.cornell.edu/education/pa
NY	CUNY York College www.york.cuny.edu/PA/index.shtml
NY	Daemen College http://daemen.edu/academics/divisionofhealthhumanservices/ physicianassistant/
NY	D'youville College www.dyc.edu/
NY	Hofstra University www.hofstra.edu/

(Continued)

State	Accredited Program
NY	Le Moyne College www.lemoyne.edu/pa
NY	Long Island University (F) www.liu.edu/
NY	Mercy College www.mercy.edu/
NY	New York Institute of Technology http://iris.nyit.edu/hpbls/pas
NY	Pace University www.pace.edu/dyson/paprogram
NY	Rochester Institute of Technology www.rit.edu/
NY	St. John's University (formerly SVCMC) www.stjohns.edu/academics/undergraduate/pharmacy/programs/pa
NY	Stony Brook University http://healthtechnology.stonybrookmedicine.edu/programs/pa/ elpa/welcome
NY	SUNY Downstate Medical Center www.downstate.edu/
NY	SUNY Upstate Medical Center www.upstate.edu/chp/programs/pa/
NY	Touro College‡ (Bay Shore) (D) www.touro.edu/
NY	Touro College (Manhattan) www.touro.edu/shs
NY	Wagner College www.wagner.edu/
OH	OH - Baldwin Wallace University (provisional†) www.bw.edu/academics/hpe/programs/physician-assistant/
OH	Cuyahoga Community College/Cleveland State University www.tri-c.edu/programs/physicianassistant/Pages/default.aspx
OH	Kettering College www.kcma.edu/

State	Accredited Program
OH	Marietta College www.marietta.edu/graduate/PA
OH	Ohio Dominican University (provisional[†]) www.ohiodominican.edu/pa/
OH	University of Toledo www.utoledo.edu/
OH	University of Mount Union www.muc.edu/pa
OH	University of Findlay www.findlay.edu/academics/colleges/cohp/academicprograms/ graduate/PHAS/default.htm
OK	University of Oklahoma, Oklahoma City www.ouhsc.edu/
OK	University of Oklahoma, Tulsa http://tulsa.ou.edu/pa/index.htm
OR	Oregon Health and Science University www.ohsu.edu/pa
OR	Pacific University www.pacificu.edu/
PA	Arcadia University (D) www.arcadia.edu/
PA	Chatham University (probation*) www.chatham.edu/departments/healthmgmt/graduate/pa/index.cfm
PA	Desales University www.desales.edu/default.aspx?pageid=331
PA	Drexel University www.drexel.edu/physAsst/programs/physicianAssistant/
PA	Duquesne University www.duq.edu/healthsciences
PA	Gannon University www.gannon.edu/
PA	King's College http://departments.kings.edu/paprog/

(Continued)

State	Accredited Program
PA	Lock Haven University (D) http://gradprograms.lhup.edu/pa/
PA	Marywood University www.marywood.edu/pa-program/
PA	Misericordia University (provisional[†]) www.misericordia.edu/misericordia_pg.cfm?subcat_id=108&page_id=990
PA	Salus University (formerly Pennsylvania College of Optometry) www.salus.edu/physicianAssistant/index.html
PA	Pennsylvania College of Technology www.pct.edu/schools/hs/pa/
PA	Philadelphia College of Osteopathic Medicine www.pcom.edu/
PA	Philadelphia University www.philau.edu/
PA	Saint Francis University www.francis.edu/
PA	Seton Hill University http://paprogram.setonhill.edu/
PA	University of Pittsburgh www.shrs.pitt.edu/pa/
PA	University of the Sciences of Philadelphia (provisional[†]) www.physicianassistant.usciences.edu/physician-assistant-studies/physician-assistant-studies-overview
SC	Medical University of South Carolina www.musc.edu/chp/pa
SD	University of South Dakota www.usd.edu/pa
TN	Bethel University[‡] www.bethelu.edu/bethelpa/
TN	Lincoln Memorial www.lmunet.edu/DCOM/pa/index.htm

State	Accredited Program
TN	Christian Brothers University (provisional[†]) www.cbu.edu/cbu/Admissions/GraduatePrograms/MSPAS/index.htm
TN	South College www.southcollegetn.edu/physician_assistant/main.htm
TN	Trevecca Nazarene University www.trevecca.edu/adult-education/graduate-programs/ physician-assistant/
TX	Baylor College of Medicine www.bcm.edu/pap
TX	Interservice www.cs.amedd.army.mil/ipap/
TX	Texas Tech University www.ttuhsc.edu/sah
TX	University of North Texas HS Center at Fort Worth www.hsc.unt.edu/education/PASP/
TX	University of Texas HS Center at San Antonio (D) www.uthscsa.edu/
TX	University of Texas Medical Branch at Galveston www.sahs.utmb.edu/pas/
TX	University of Texas Pan American www.panam.edu/dept/pasp
TX	University of Texas SW School of Health Professions www8.utsouthwestern.edu/utsw/cda/dept48945/files/54102.html
UT	University of Utah http://medicine.utah.edu/UPAP/
VA	Eastern Virginia Medical School www.evms.edu/evms-school-of-health-professions/physician- assistant.html
VA	James Madison University www.jmu.edu/healthsci/paweb
VA	Jefferson College of Health Sciences (formerly CHS) www.jchs.edu/page.php/prmID/382

(Continued)

State	Accredited Program
VA	Shenandoah University www.su.edu/pa
WA	University of Washington (D) www.medex.washington.edu/
WI	Carroll University (provisional[†]) www.carrollu.edu/gradprograms/physasst/default.asp
WI	Concorida University (provisional[†]) www.cuw.edu/programs/physicianassistant/index.html
WI	Marquette University www.marquette.edu/chs/pa/index.shtml
WI	University of Wisconsin La Crosse www.uwlax.edu/pastudies
WI	University of Wisconsin Madison www.physicianassistant.wisc.edu/index.htm
WV	Alderson-Broaddus College[‡] (provisional[†]) http://ab.edu/academics/master-science-physician-assistant-studies
WV	Mountain State University www.mountainstate.edu/
WV	University of Charleston (provisional[†]) www.ucwv.edu/PA/
WV	West Liberty University (provisional[†]) www.westliberty.edu/physician-assistant/

[*]"Accreditation-Probation" is a temporary status of accreditation assigned when a program does not meet the *Standards* and when the capability of the program to provide an acceptable educational experience for its students is threatened. Once placed on probation, programs that still fail to comply with accreditation requirements in a timely manner, as specified by the ARC-PA, may be scheduled for a focused site visit and/or risk having their accreditation withdrawn. A program on probation must provide clear evidence of progress toward improving the program by its next ARC-PA review. The maximum period of probation is two years.

[†]"Accreditation-Provisional" is an accreditation status granted for a limited, defined period of time to a new program that has demonstrated its preparedness to initiate a program in accordance with the *Standards*.

[‡]Indicates that a program was closed for a period of time since being first accredited.

(D) indicates that accreditation incorporates one or more distant campuses.

(F) indicates that a program may have a focused visit prior to its next ARC-PA review.

Physician Assistant Residencies

This information below is provided by the Accreditation Review Commission on Education for the Physician Assistant (ARC-PA) at www.arc-pa.com/postgrad_programs/acc_clinical_programs.html and was last updated on April 12, 2013.

State	Accredited Program
AZ	Mayo Clinic Postgraduate PA ENT Residency www.mayo.edu/mshs/pa-otorhino-sct.html
AZ	Mayo Clinic Postgraduate PA Hospital Internal Medicine Residency www.mayo.edu/mshs/pa-him-sct.html
CA	Arrowhead Orthopedics Postgraduate PA Orthopedics Residency www.arrowheadortho.com/pa.htm
IA	University of Iowa Postgraduate PA Emergency Medicine Residency www.uihealthcare.org/GME/ResProgHome.aspx?pageid=231957&taxid=226453
MD	Johns Hopkins Hospital Department of Surgery Postgraduate PA Surgical Residency www.hopkinsmedicine.org/surgery/education/pa_residency/index.html
NC	Duke University Medical Center Postgraduate PA Surgical Residency http://surgery.duke.edu/education-and-training/residency-programs/pa-surgical-residency-program

(Continued)

State	Accredited Program
TX	MD Anderson Cancer Center Postgraduate PA Program in Oncology www.mdanderson.org/prof_education/medical_ed/display.cfm?id=7E9D932E-2515-11D5-811100508B603A14&method=displayFull&pn=305D145F-133C-4348-807311A61D8890D5
VA	Naval Medical Center (Portsmouth) Postgraduate PA Program in Orthopedics www.navy.com/navy/careers/healthcare/clinical-care/physician-assistant/?campaign=search_Reprise/Bing/Physician+Assistant+Navy/navy+pa+program&sid=navy+pa+program

Glossary

ablation	Surgical destruction of a body part and its ability to function.
acanthosis	A thickening of one of the five layers of the skin, the layer known as the *prickle-cell layer*.
adrenaline	A hormone secreted by the adrenal medulla in response to physical or mental stress that causes increased heart rate and increased blood pressure. Also called *epinephrine*.
amyotrophic lateral sclerosis (ALS)	A progressive degenerative disease of the lateral columns of the spinal cord leading to weakness, paralysis, and death. Also called *Lou Gehrig's disease*.
anhedonia	Uncharacteristic loss of pleasure doing activities that are normally pleasurable.
ankylosing spondylitis	Arthritis of the spine that causes the vertebrae to fuse and become inflexible.
anticoagulate	Any agent that prevents the formation of blood clots.
aortic dissection	A tear in the middle wall of the aorta leading to an aortic aneurysm.
arrhythmia	Irregular rhythm of the heart.
arterial blood gas (ABG)	The measure of oxygen and carbon dioxide levels and pH in a sample of blood taken from an artery.
arthropathies	Any disease relating to the joints.
arthroscopy	Surgical examination of a joint in which an arthroscope is inserted into a joint.
audiogram	The graphic result of a hearing test.
aura	Symptoms such as flashing lights, numbness, or weakness that signal the onset of a migraine headache or a seizure.

autograft	An organ or tissue grafted into a new position in the body of the individual from which it came; autotransplant.
autoimmune	Denoting an immune-system response by the body against one or more of its own tissues.
azoospermia	The absence of live spermotozoa in the semen.
barium swallow	A series of x-rays of the esophagus, stomach, and small intestines after the patient has swallowed barium sulfate.
benign	Not malignant; used especially with cancers to indicate that they are not invasive and spreading.
body mass index (BMI)	A general measure of nutritional status, giving a general measurement of the amount of fat in a person's body, calculated by dividing the person's weight in kilograms (kg) by the square of his or her height in meters (m^2).
brachytherapy	Radiation therapy performed close to the site being eradiated, for example by implantation of radioactive seeds into a prostate tumor.
bradycardia	A slow heart rate, less than 60 beats per minute.
breech presentation	A position in which the fetus is in the birth canal with the feet or buttocks closest to the cervix; labor often ends with a cesarean section.
calculi	A small stonelike mass of material in a body cavity or organ, usually formed of mineral salts and typically found in the urinary bladder or gallbladder.
cardiopulmonary bypass	A surgical procedure to divert blood that is blocked from returning to the heart.
catarrh	Inflammation or infection of the membranes of the nose or throat, usually involving overproduction of mucus.
catatonic	Of, pertaining to, or characteristic of catatonia (a state of rigidity or bizarre movements usually associated with mental disorder such as schizophrenia).
cautery	Any substance or instrument used in cauterizing. (The destruction of tissue with a chemical, electricity, or hot or cold instrumentation, usually to stop excessive bleeding or seal off a wound.

cholecystitis	Inflammation of the gallbladder.
chronotropic	Affecting the tuning or rate of something, such as a heartbeat.
claudication	Limping, frequently due to insufficient blood flow (oxygen delivery) to the leg muscles.
colposcopy	Examination of the vagina using a colposcope.
comedones	A small plug of sebum blocking the duct of a sebaceous gland especially on the face. Also called a *blackhead*.
compartment syndrome	A condition in which there is swelling and inflammation isolated to one section of the body, such as an arm or a leg, causing compression of blood supply and nerves, usually requiring immediate surgery.
computed tomography (CT)	An x-ray technique using several x-ray beams in different positions and computer processing to produce cross-sectional images of the body. Also called *computerized (axial) tomography*.
conjunctivitis	Inflammation of the conjunctiva, commonly called *pink eye*.
convulsion	A violent spasm or seizure.
corneal abrasion	A scratch on the cornea.
coronary artery bypass grafting (CABG)	A surgical procedure in which a new blood vessel (vein or artery) is grafted onto the heart to bridge a blockage of an artery.
crackles	Short, rough inspiratory sounds produced by inflamed or fluid-overloaded lungs, as heard through a stethoscope.
Crohn's disease	An inflammatory disease of the digestive system characterized by intestinal ulcers, abdominal pain, diarrhea, vomiting, fever, and weight loss.
cryotherapy	The use of cold temperatures to treat injuries of disease.
cystocele	Hernia of the bladder through the vaginal wall.
cystoscope	A thin tubular instrument with a light used to examine the interior of the bladder.
cystoscopy	Examination of the bladder using a cystoscope.

cystostomy	Surgical creation of a hole in the bladder to drain urine while allowing surgery on the urethra to heal.
cystourethro-gram	X-ray image of the bladder and urethra made after a contrast medium has been injected.
debridement	Removal of dead and dying tissue from a wound or burn to help the healing process.
degenerative disk	The gradual weakening and compression of a vertebral disk.
delirium	An altered mental state that includes confusion, disorientation, and hallucinations and may have either a physical or emotional cause.
dementia	The progressive loss of cognitive functions, usually associated with old age or a brain disease.
demyelination	Loss of myelin from the nerve sheath, causing a slowing of conduction and associated with certain diseases, such as multiple sclerosis.
dermatome	A cutting instrument used for removing thin slices of skin.
desquamation	The shedding of scaling of the outer layer of skin.
DEXA scan	The image or data produced by a special x-ray machine used to measure bone density.
dialysis	The process of cleaning the blood by passing it through a special machine (hemodialysis) or by filling the peritoneum with a cleansing solution (peritoneal dialysis)
disk herniation	A rupture of the connective tissue between two or more vertebral bones or a bulging of the tissue from the interior of a disk.
diskectomy	The surgical removal of a disk from between the vertebrae.
diuretics	An agent that increases the production and excretion of urine.
dysphagia	Difficulty swallowing.
ecchymosis	A discoloration of the skin or mucus membrane caused by blood escaping from ruptured blood vessels; informally called a *black and blue mark*. Also called a *bruise*.

echocardio-gram (ECHO)	The record obtained by echocardiography.
echocardiogra-phy	A technique of monitoring the heart that uses ultrasound to take two-dimensional images of the heart both at rest and during exercise. It can demonstrate blood flow direction, such as with a leaky valve.
effusion	The seeping of fluid into a body cavity or tissue.
ejection fraction (EF)	During a heartbeat, the blood pumped out of a filled ventricle when the heart contracts, expressed as a percentage of ventricular volume.
electrocautery	An instrument for passing a high-frequency current through a local area of tissue.
embolus	A blood clot or small particle of bone marrow fat that travels in the bloodstream and lodges in a smaller vessel, obstructing the flow of blood.
endoscopy	The visual inspection of a body cavity or canal with an endoscope.
enuresis	Urinary incontinence, especially bedwetting at night.
epistaxis	Bleeding from the nose.
escharotomy	Incision into an eschar. (Eschar: Scab formed from cautery.)
fascia	A sheet of connective tissue that envelopes part of the body underneath the skin; it covers or binds muscles together and supports soft tissue structures in the body, such as organs.
fiber optic	The transmission of light signals through glass fibers, used in imaging.
fibromyalgia	A syndrome characterized by chronic musculoskeletal pain and stiffness with no detectable inflammation, tenderness at specific sites of the body (trigger points), fatigue, and severe sleep disturbance; the exact cause is unknown.
fibrosis	Formation of extra fibrous tissue as a reactive process or in repair of something rather than as part of normal tissue building.

fistula	An abnormal duct or passageway leading from an organ to the body surface or to another organ, usually resulting from an injury or disease.
fluoroscopy	Examination of the body using a fluoroscope.
fluroscope	A device containing a screen covered with a fluorescent substance that allows the observer to see the pattern revealed by x-rays, used for viewing structures within the body.
fundoplication	A surgical technique that fortifies the barrier between the stomach and the lower esophagus to prevent acid reflux.
gestational diabetes mellitus	A form of diabetes mellitus that appears during pregnancy and usually disappears after delivery; it can predispose the mother to later type 2 diabetes.
glomerulonephritis	A kidney disease characterized by inflammation of the renal glomeruli.
grand mal seizure	A type of epileptic seizure characterized by two phases, in which first the body becomes rigid and then starts to jerk uncontrollably.
Hashimoto's thyroiditis	An autoimmune disease of the thyroid gland in which lymphocytes infiltrate the thyroid, characterized by goiter, inflammation of the thyroid, and hypothyroidism. Also called *struma lymphomatosa*.
hematuria	The presence of blood in the urine.
hemodialysis	A type of dialysis in which waste material and toxic substances are filtered out of the blood using a dialysis machine.
hemoglobin A1c	A blood test to measure the percentage of hemoglobin bound with glucose to monitor treatment of diabetes mellitus. Also called *glycosylated hemoglobin test*.
hemoglobin/ hematocrit (H/H)	Hemoglobin: The oxygen-carrying protein pigment in red blood cells measured in grams/100 mL. Hematocrit: The percentage of red blood cells in a blood sample after centrifugation.
hemoglobinopathy	Any disease characterized by the presence of abnormal hemoglobin in the blood.

hemophilia	Any of a group of diseases characterized by delayed blood clotting.
hemoptysis	Coughing up blood from the respiratory tract.
hemorrhage	Severe excessive bleeding.
hemostasis	The stoppage of bleeding or blood flow.
hidradenitis	Infection or inflammation of the sweat glands.
hirsutism	Abnormal excessive hair growth, especially in women.
hydronephrosis	Condition with accumulation of excess urine in the kidneys due to obstruction of urine outflow.
hyperemesis	Excessive vomiting.
hyperemesis gravidarum	Excessive nausea and vomiting during pregnancy, resulting in dehydration and acidosis.
ileus	Obstruction or blockage of the ileum.
immunocom- promised	Impairment or insufficient development of immune response.
immunoglobu- lin (Ig)	Any in the family of glycoproteins (molecules consisting of a simple sugar attached to an amino acid) that function as antibodies in immune response.
immunosup- presive agent	An agent that slows immune response to prevent the body's natural rejection of grafts or transplants.
insulin	A hormone secreted by the pancreas that regulates gylcogen storage in the liver, facilitates the entry of glucose into cells, and helps regulate carbohydrate and fat metabolism, especially in converting glucose to glycogen; also produced as a medication for people with diabetes.
insulin pump	A portable device that infuses insulin continuously, with additional doses to cover meals, used by people with diabetes to control blood sugar levels.
insulin resistance	A state of reduced effectiveness of insulin in lowering blood sugar levels.
interdisciplinary	Involving two or more specialties in medicine or science.

jaundice	A yellowish discoloration of the skin or whites of the eyes due to high levels of bilirubin in the blood.
keratolytic	Of, relating to, or causing keratolysis.
ketoacidosis	Acidosis caused by the excessive production of ketones or ketone bodies, as in uncontrolled diabetes or starvation.
ketone	A by-product of fat metabolism.
ketosis	An increase of ketone bodies in the blood.
kyphoscoliosis	A condition in which kyphosis and scoliosis are present.
kyphosis	Abnormal outward curvature of the thoracic spine resulting in a hunchback appearance.
laminectomy	Surgical procedure in which the laminae (bony arches) of one or more vertebrae are removed in order to alleviate compression of the spinal cord.
laminotomy	The surgical division of a vertebral lamina.
laparoscope	An endoscope (fiber-optic instrument with an illuminated tube) designed for examining the abdominal cavity.
laxity	Degree of freedom of movement of a joint.
lethargic	State of dullness, extreme drowsiness, sluggishness, apathy.
lumbar puncture (LP)	The insertion of a needle into the space between two lumbar vertebrae, usually the third and fourth, to withdraw spinal fluid for examination and sometimes to inject medication. Also called *spinal puncture, spinal tap*.
lymphadenopathy	Any abnormal or diseased condition of the lymph nodes.
menorrhagia	Abnormally heavy or prolonged menstrual flow.
microanastamosis	A functioning link between tubular structures.
myelofibrosis	Proliferation of fibroblastic cells in bone marrow causing anemia and sometimes enlargement of the spleen and liver.
myleopathy	Disease of the spinal cord.

myringotomy	Surgical puncturing of the eardrum to release fluid.
nephrolithiasis	Condition of having calculi (stones) in the kidney.
nephrostomy	A surgical incision into a kidney.
neurogenic	Originating in nerve tissue or in a nerve.
neuropathy	A painful condition usually of feet in which a disorder of sensory nerves causes hypersensitivity to tactile stimuli; often present in diabetes.
neutropenia	Disorder with abnormally low number of neutrophils in the bloodstream.
nocturia	Excessive urination at night.
orchalgia	Pain in the testicle.
orthostatic hypotension	A drop in blood pressure on rapid change of position, such as standing up.
osteomyelitis	An inflammation or infection of bone marrow and bone.
osteotomy	Surgical incision into a bone.
palpitations	A sudden sensation that the heart is throbbing irregularly or harder or faster than normal, with the pulse going over 100 beats per minute.
Papanicolaou's stain (Pap)	A chemical preparation used to stain specimens for microscopic examination, as in the Pap test.
papule	A small, firm bump on the skin, often inflamed.
paracentesis	Surgical insertion of a needle or other instrument into a body cavity, especially the abdomen, to withdraw fluid from it.
paraplegia	Paralysis of the legs and the lower part of the torso.
patent ductus arteriosus	Failure of the ductus arteriosous to close after birth.
pedunculated	Having a stalk that attaches a growth to skin or body tissue.
percutaneous	Administered through the skin by injection or a transdermal patch.

perforation	An abnormal opening in the wall of an organ or vessel or through a body part.
pericardium	The membrane that covers the heart in the beginnings of the large blood vessels. It consists of two layers: the visceral and parietal layers.
petechial hemorrhage	Bleeding into the skin from the small blood vessels that cause petechiae. Also called *punctate hemorrhage*.
phlebotomy	Puncturing a vein to draw blood.
plasma	The fluid part of blood, consisting of water, proteins, salts, nutrients, clotting factors, and hormones.
pleurectomy	The surgical removal of a part of the pleura.
***Pneumocystis carinii* pneumonia (PCP)**	The former classification of the species of protozoan that causes *Pneumocystis* pneumonia in immunosuppressed patients. Also called *Pneumocystis pneumonia*.
polycistic ovary syndrome	A condition in women marked by lack of ovulation, acne, obesity, and excess body hair.
porphyria	Any of a group of usually inherited disorders in the production of heme (the part of hemoglobin that carries the oxygen).
postvoid residual	Urine that remains in the bladder after urination.
prophylactic	An agent, such as a medicinal preparation, that prevents the spread of disease.
psoriasis	A common, chronic skin disorder that flares up periodically and is marked by red, scale-covered patches of skin, especially on bony parts of the body such as the knees, elbows, scalp, and trunk; may be accompanied by a type of arthritis.
pulmonary artery (PA)	The blood vessel that carries deoxygenated blood from the right ventricle of the heart to the lungs, where it becomes oxygenated and returns to the heart. After it leaves the heart, the artery divides into two branches, called the right and left pulmonary arteries, which lead to the right and left lungs.

pulmonary artery catheter	A small balloon-tipped catheter inserted through the heart into the pulmonary artery for the purpose of measuring cardiac output and pulmonary artery pressure.
pulmonary hypertension	High blood pressure in the pulmonary artery, which carries blood from the right ventricle of the heart to the lungs; may be primary or secondary to another disease. Also called *pulmonary heart disease, pulmonary arterial hypertension*.
pyrexia	Fever.
pyuria	Having pus in the urine; usually indicating a urinary tract infection.
radiculopathy	Any disease of the nerve roots.
rectocele	Protrusion of the rectum into the vagina.
repolarization	Restoration of a polarized state across a membrane, with positive charges on the outer surface and negative charges on the inner surface.
retinal detachment	Visual impairment in which the retina has separated from the choroid.
retinopathy	Any noninflammatory degenerative condition of the retina.
retroperitoneal	Located behind the peritoneum, as are the kidneys, ureters, bladder, uterus, etc.
sarcoidosis	A disease with no known cause characterized by firm, grainy, or small, nodular lesions in the liver, lungs, shin, and lymph nodes.
sarcoma	A malignant tumor formed in connective tissue.
scabies	A contagious skin disease caused by *Sarcoptes scabiei*, known as the itch mite, characterized by intense persistent itching.
scald	To burn with hot liquid or steam.
scleroderma	A pathologic thickening and hardening of the skin.
scoliosis	Abnormal lateral curvature of the spine.
scopy	Suffix meaning viewing, seeing, or observing: for example, endoscopy.

sepsis	The presence of pathogenetic organisms or their toxins in the bloodstream.
sickle-cell disease	A severe type of inherited anemia in which an abnormal hemoglobin molecule causes the red blood cell to take a crescent shape when in low-oxygen conditions; usually only found in races indigenous to areas where malaria is prevalent. Called *SS disease*, meaning that the gene comes from both parents; found most commonly in African Americans.
silver nitrate	A powerful antiseptic used topically, such as immediately after birth in the eyes (to prevent gonorrheal ophthalmitis), to prevent or cure certain infections.
slit lamp	Examination of the eye using a device with a high-intensity light focused on the eye structures.
spasm	A sudden and strong involuntary muscle contracture.
spirometry	Measuring the amount of air entering and exiting the lungs using a spirometer.
stem cell	An undifferentiated (unspecialized) cell that can grow into any one of the body's cell types.
stupor	Impaired consciousness marked by reduced responsiveness to stimuli.
subarachnoid	Space between the arachnoid and the pia mater in the tissue surrounding and protecting the brain and spinal cord.
subdural hematoma	Hematoma beneath the dura mater; may apply extreme pressure to the cerebral cortex after head trauma, especially in the elderly; often a surgical emergency.
syncope	A brief loss of consciousness caused by a sudden drop in blood pressure or failure of cardiac systole, resulting in cerebral hypoxia. Also called *fainting*.
syndrome of inappropriate antidiuretic hormone (SIADH)	A condition seen with certain diseases (particularly certain types of cancers) with the inappropriate secretion of antidiuretic hormone resulting in water retention, inhibition of urine excretion, and secondary symptoms such as nausea or convulsions.
tetraparesis	Weakness of all four limbs (arms and legs), usually the result of a spinal cord injury or stroke. Also called *quadriparesis*.

thoracentesis	Removal of fluid from the chest by puncturing for therapeutic or diagnostic purposes. Also called *pleurocentesis, thoracocentesis.*
thoracotomy	A surgical incision of the chest wall.
thrombectomy	Surgical removal of a blood clot.
thrombosis	Formation or presence of blood clot in a blood vessel.
tracheostomy	Surgical opening of the trachea, through the neck, to facilitate breathing.
transient ischemic attack (TIA)	Temporary blockage of a cerebral blood vessel resulting in dizziness and numbness on one side of the body or temporary loss of vision. Informally called a *ministroke.*
trichotillomania	The compulsion to pull out one's hair; considered to be a psychosomatic symptom.
tympanic membrane	The membrane that separates the external ear from the middle ear.
varices	Plural of varix.
varix	A distended, misshapen blood or lymph vessel.
vasodilator	Something, such as a medication, that causes vasodilation and lowering of blood pressure.
vasopressor	Something that causes vasoconstriction, thereby raising blood pressure.
vericocele	Distended or swollen veins in the spermatic cord or in the uterus or ovaries.
vertex	The top of something, especially the crown of the head.
vertigo	The sensation that oneself or one's surroundings are spinning.
vital capacity (VC)	The maximum amount of air that can be exhaled from the lungs after inhaling the greatest possible amount of air.
Von Willebrand disease	A hereditary disorder marked by a tendency to bleed extensively, such as after surgery or during menstruation, and by various clotting irregularities in the blood.

whooping cough	A highly infectious childhood respiratory disease caused by the bacterium *Bordatella pertussis* with spasmodic coughing and deep inhalations. Also called *pertussis*.
xanthochromic	Yellowish in color.
xenograft	Tissue taken from an animal of one species and used as a graft, often temporarily, in an animal of another species.

All terms/definitions are from: McGraw-Hill's Medical Dictionary for Allied Health by Breskin, Dumith, Pearsons and Seeman Copyright 2008